Preface • L

Not all organizations need to be an HRO. However, organizations that deal with "low probability, high consequence" events – incidents that are extremely unlikely but should they occur, have consequences that would be severe to the organization – really have no choice but to become an HRO.

We at B&W Pantex, because of our unique mission and service to our Country, must strive to become an HRO. Our manufacturing operations require a practical approach to high reliability operations that is deployable, sustainable, and effective. One trait that every HRO needs to focus on is institutional learning; our Causal Factor Analysis process addresses that need. We developed this practical guide based on our experience to address the special considerations of becoming an HRO. The practices are stated in universal terms and will help other high-hazard operations pursue the same goal.

Regardless of the need to be an HRO, every organization in today's society must grow and sustain a healthy safety culture that serves the operations of the organization. The first step in this regard is to treat safety not as a priority; but as a core value that is integrated into everything the organization does. This is the premise of the approach to safety reflected in this guide. Every organization, regardless of its pursuit to become an HRO, will see value in using this guide to improve their safety culture and attain safe operations.

J. G. Meyer, CSP
President & General Manager, B&W Pantex

HIGH RELIABILITY ORGANIZATION, PANTEX CORPORATION

Copyright, 2008, Babcock & Wilcox Technical Services Pantex LLC (B&W Pantex)

This manuscript was authored by B&W Pantex, under Contract Number DE-AC04-00AL66620, with the U.S. Department of Energy. The United States Government retains and the recipients, by accepting these materials, acknowledges that the United States Government retains a non-exclusive, paid-up, irrevocable, world-wide license to publish or reproduce the published form of this manuscript, or allow others to do so, for United States Government purposes.

This document was produced by B&W Pantex
P.O. Box 30020
Amarillo, TX 79120
(806) 477-3000
Managing and Operating Contractor for the
U.S. Department of Energy
Pantex Plant, Amarillo, Texas
under
U.S. Government Contract DE-AC04-00AL66620
ISBN 0-16-083144-7

ACKNOWLEDGEMENTS

No text ever written is the product of only one person's efforts, and certainly this one was no different. This collection of information would never have become a text without the research, personal experiences, and ideas of many co-workers at B&W Pantex. Their support, encouragement and feedback provided the impetus to finish this text. During the often interrupted evolution of this text, many debts have accumulated, only a few of which there is space to acknowledge here: Linda Caufman, Cathie Harris, Jane Lincoln, Mike Reaka, and Kim Leffew.

Special thanks to Bill Corcoran, NSRC Corporation, who provided a great deal of information on safety culture and the practical applications of Causal Factors Analysis and Earl Carnes/DOE, who provided many thought-provoking discussions on the topic of high reliability organizations and safety culture.

Special thanks also to Anna Stickrod, who patiently edited these texts numerous times to achieve the desired level of quality.

Contents

Letter from Plant Manager	1
Acknowledgements	2
Acronyms and Abbreviations	6

**Chapter 1 Understanding What it Means
to be a High Reliability Organization** **7**
The Systems Perspective: How Organizations Function as Systems 11
What is a System Accident? 11
High-Hazard Operations: The Risk Factor 16
A Practical Systems Approach to High Reliability: Four
    Guiding Practices 23
The HRO Journey: What You Should Know Before You Go 32

**Chapter 2 Knowing Where You Are Headed: How to Manage
the System** **37**
Manage the System, Not the Parts 38
Making the Practices Work: A Mindful Approach 44

**Chapter 3 Transforming to an HRO: How to Develop a
Guiding Strategy** **53**
A Systems Approach to Strategic Planning 54
The McKinsey 7S Approach: Seven Elements to Guide
    Your HRO Journey 58
Using the Four HRO Practices to Inform Strategy Development 68
How to Apply the 7S Approach: An Illustrative Example 68

**Chapter 4 Break the Chain Between Threat and Hazard:
A Safety System Framework** **81**
Common Pitfalls that Can Lead to System Accidents 82
Deploy the Break-the-Chain Safety Framework 96
Evaluate the Operation of the Safety System 113
Systematically Adjust Processes 113

Chapter 5 Fostering a Culture of Reliability **121**
What is a Culture of Reliability? 122
How to Foster a Strong Culture of Reliability 126

Chapter 6 Learning and Adapting as an Organization:

The Feedback Loop   **131**

Generating Decision-making Information: A Tiered Approach
to Organizational Learning   133

Integrate and Interpret Feedback to Enable Better Decision Making   150

Refine the HRO System: Apply a Systems Approach to Reduce
Variability   153

Chapter 7 Evaluating Your Organization's Culture of Reliability:

Determine the Effectiveness of the HRO Practices   **159**

Characterize Your Organization's Culture of Reliability   160

Evaluate Your Organization's Culture of Reliability   166

What If My Organization's Culture Is Not Healthy?   184

Chapter 8 Wrapping it Up: What You Should Take Away

from this Guide   **187**

The Importance of a System Approach   188

Pointers to Help You Achieve and Maintain High Reliability
Operations   192

References   **195**

Notes   **201**

Index   **203**

Figures

Figure 1-1. System versus Individual Accidents   15

Figure 1-2. Redundant Systems: Barriers Between Employees
and Plant   21

Figure 1-3. The Four HRO Practices and Their Relationship
to the Theory of Profound Knowledge   27

Figure 1-4. Roadmap to High Reliability Operations   35

Figure 2-1. Sustaining Characteristics of Mindful HROs   47

Figure 3-1. HRO Transformation Process   54

Figure 3-2. McKinsey 7S Approach for HRO Transformation   56

Figure 3-3. The 7S Elements Applied to the HRO Practices   58

Figure 4-1. The Break-the-Chain Framework   83

Figure 4-2. Human Error Performance Modes   87

Figure 4-3. Defeating Defense-in-Depth: Effect of Active
and Latent Errors on Barriers   92

Figure 4-4. Organizational Causes of Accidents   95
Figure 4-5. The Break-the-Chain Framework and its Relationship
    to the HRO Practices   97
Figure 4-6. TWIN Analysis Matrix   104
Figure 5-1. Schein Levels of Culture   124
Figure 6-1. The Break-the-Chain Framework and the
    Tiered Approach to Organizational Learning   135
Figure 6-2. Barrier Analysis Matrix   139
Figure 6-3. Causal Factors Analysis to Determine
    Organizational Weaknesses   144
Figure 6-4. Output of Causal Factors Analysis to Evaluate
    HRO Attributes   145
Figure 6-5. Causal Factors Analysis Flowchart   148
Figure 6-6. Why We Care About Safety Culture   157
Figure 7-1. Characterization of Safety Culture   162
Figure 7-2. Culture of Reliability   167

Tables

Table 2-1. The Mindful Organization: How the Attributes
    of Mindfulness Relate to the Four HRO Practices   48
Table 3-1. Company Alpha Strategies, Measures, and Targets   79
Table 6-1. Common Organizational Weaknesses   154
Table 7-1. Actions, Lines of Inquiry, and Suggested Metrics   172
Table 8-1. Relationship Between Deming's Theory of Profound
    Knowledge and the Four HRO Practices   189

Acronyms and Abbreviations

CFA   Causal Factors Analysis

DOE   United States Department of Energy

ECAQ   extraneous conditions adverse to quality

HRO   high reliability organization

IT   Information Technology

INPO   Institute of Nuclear Power Operations

LTBL   lessons to be learned

PDCA   planning, doing, checking, and acting

SMART   specific

                   measurable

                   agreed-to

                   realistic, and

                   time-bound

TWIN   An analysis tool that focuses on task demands, work environment, individual capabilities, and human nature as the four types of human error precursors

Chapter 1

Chapter 1

Understanding What it Means to be a High Reliability Organization

This chapter answers the following questions:

- What is a high reliability organization (HRO)?

- My high-hazard operation has an excellent safety record—does that mean it is an HRO?

- Why should my organization strive to become an HRO?

- What is a system accident and how does it differ from other types of accidental events I am trying to prevent?

- Is my high-hazard operation more prone to system accidents than other operations?

- Why is a systems approach necessary to prevent the accident my organization fears most?

- What are four organizational practices that will enable my organization to nourish and support high reliability operations?

Are you involved in managing a high-hazard operation? If so, you have probably asked yourself the question: "How can I protect the operation I manage, which involves hazardous materials and is operated by fallible individuals, from catastrophe?" You have probably heard the term *high reliability organization* (HRO) and know that it represents an approach that aims to address this question. But what exactly is an HRO?

> **Systems Failures Can Lead To Catastrophe**
>
> "Some types of system failures are so punishing that they must be avoided at almost any cost. These classes of events are seen as so harmful that they disable the organization, radically limiting its capacity to pursue its goal, and could lead to its own destruction."
>
> *(LaPorte and Consolini, 1991, p. 27)*

To paraphrase Karlene Roberts (2003), a professor in the Haas School of Business at the University of California at Berkeley and a pioneer in HRO theory[1]:

An HRO is an organization that conducts relatively error-free operations over a long period of time, making consistently good decisions that result in high quality and reliable operations.

Inherent in this definition are the concepts of reliability and safety, which have distinct connotations. Reliability indicates consistency and trustworthiness, and suggests merit. When we call an organization reliable, we typically mean that it provides dependable, high-quality goods or services. As a consumer or customer, we feel sure that we will obtain the same excellent results each time we deal with this organization. Safety is a condition of being relatively free of danger from hazards. When we are safe, we are protected against physical, social, financial, political, occupational, or other types of harm. Thus, an HRO must provide excellent, dependable goods or services and—at the same time—make sure its employees, the environment, and the public are protected against harm from the hazardous operations under its control.

Most high-hazard operations are able to operate successfully for long periods of time without major accidents. For example, commercial airlines have an excellent safety record: the chances of being involved in an aircraft accident are about 1 in 11 million, as opposed to a 1 in 5,000 chance of being killed in an automobile accident (Nielson). Does this mean that major airline companies operate as HROs? Or, perhaps your organization is a nuclear power plant with an unblemished safety record, which has supplied reliable power to a growing consumer base for more than 25 years. Does this make you an HRO?

No. Our contention is that an organization is not an HRO unless it has both an excellent safety and production record and it strives, on a daily basis, to implement and sustain practices that will ensure both safety and reliability. In fact, we would argue that your organization is probably more vulnerable to a major accident if it relies solely on its exemplary safety record (e.g., low total reportable accidents or low lost time rates). Why? Because it is human nature to grow complacent about those aspects of our life or work that we think we have under control. An excellent safety record may lull an organization into believing its operations are fail-safe; as a result, managers and employees may divert attention to other areas of the operation. A condition known as *practical drift* may creep into daily operations; employees may unintentionally veer away from the controls meant to ensure system safety. For example, operators may begin to use short cuts instead of following standard operating procedures, or you, a manager, might assume that it's okay not to fill a position in your division because "Joe's group covers that anyway and we have never had a serious accident in that area."

Organizations tend toward practical drift not because they don't value safety, but because they feel too safe because of lack of consequence— and perhaps because the pressure from competing demands requires them to look for areas where they can save time or money (we all know the adage, "The squeaky wheel gets the grease"). On their own, these shifts in priorities may not result in major consequences. But, as the Columbia shuttle accident has shown, multiple small failures or unplanned system events can lead to catastrophe.

Why High-hazard Operations Become HROs

To become a high reliability organization is not easy; it requires a well-designed strategy, perseverance, and resources. Despite this, more and more high-hazard industries— including commercial nuclear facilities, aircraft carrier operations, commercial airlines, hospitals, nuclear weapons operations, forest service operations, and petroleum and chemical operations—are taking the plunge.

Why? Because these operations share a common trait: they cannot afford the consequences of a catastrophic failure or accident. HROs realize how devastating such an event can be and employ a systems approach to minimize both the likelihood and associated impacts of operational mishaps.

Exemplary Safety Record Does Not Immunize Against Catastrophe—The Columbia Accident Of 2003

Vibrant industrial safety programs were found in every area examined, reflecting a common interview comment: "If anything, we go overboard on safety." Industrial safety programs are highly visible: they are nearly always a topic of work center meetings and are represented by numerous safety campaigns and posters.

(p. 217)

The NASA Shuttle Logistics Depot focus on safety has been recognized as an Occupational Safety and Health Administration Star Site for its participation in the Voluntary Protection Program. After the Shuttle Logistics Depot was recertified in 2002, employees worked more than 750 days without a lost-time mishap.

(p. 218)

Finding: 10.4-1 Shuttle System industrial safety programs are in good health.

(p. 219)

(CAIB, 2003)

Can your business face or recover from the consequences of a system failure or accident?

If the answer is no, you should seriously consider aligning your organization's cultural norms and operating practices with the HRO concepts and practical approaches presented in this guide. The HRO concept involves employing a systems approach to reduce the vulnerabilities introduced due to human error (or fallibility) to avoid the unbearable consequence that could cause severe damage to an entire industry (e.g., consider how the Three Mile Island accident affected the commercial nuclear industry).

The Systems Perspective: How Organizations Function as Systems

In the context of this guide, a system refers to an organization, specifically, an organization that engages in operations that involve high-hazard processes or materials. Because an organizational system is more robust than an individual, HROs deploy systems to reduce the vulnerabilities incurred when dealing with hazardous operations.

A system is "a group of interacting, interrelated, or interdependent components that form a complex and unified whole" (Anderson and Johnson, 1997). In fact, it is this interacting, interrelated group of components that makes a system robust. Systems may be mechanical, organizational (e.g., administrative), or sociotechnical (i.e., a combination of people and technology).

According to Ludwig von Bertalanffy (1968), organizations function as open systems. This means they have continuous interactions with their environments and they act as a whole, such that a change in one element of the system affects other elements of the system. Systems tend toward a state of stability or a "lowest energy state;" open systems will never entirely achieve this state because of their continuous interaction with the external environment. They can, however, achieve a functional steady state similar to the metabolism of a living organism, which makes them resistant to change. Like living organisms, organizations also have differentiated parts that are functionally segregated from the whole, but cannot survive on their own. For example, the accounting department of an organization may institute its own policies and procedures and function independently of the operational departments, yet it could not exist without the operational aspects of the business.

Change can be initiated within an organization by the organization's own growth and development toward a desired end-state, or from external stimuli and responses. Such changes may help solve the immediate problems faced by the organization, but—without proper consideration of how these changes might affect the entire system—can lead to problems in other parts of the system. Thus, today's problems may have been unintentionally set into motion by yesterday's solutions.

What is a System Accident?

HROs aim to avoid *system accidents* through the use of organizational design and management approaches (Sagan, 1993). But what is a system accident and how does it differ from other types of events or accidents?

An accident is an occurrence that is unplanned and unforeseen. An accident may result in unfortunate consequences or not—for example, if you are driving on an icy road and your car accidentally slides into the ditch, you may be

---

The Alternative To HRO – The System Accident

Three Mile Island Nuclear Facility—1979

Bhopal, India Industrial Plant—1984

Challenger and Columbia Space Shuttles—1986 and 2003

Chernobyl Nuclear Facility—1986

Exxon Valdez Spill—1989

Texas City BP Explosion—2005

Next?

Characteristics Of Systems

- All parts of a system are needed for it to function. If parts can be removed and the system still functions, it is a collection, not a system.

- Parts must be arranged in a certain way to carry out the purpose. If they can be combined at random, it is not a system.

- Systems have specific purposes within a larger scheme. They cannot be combined or divided and stay identical to the original.

- Systems seek stability through interaction, feedback, and adjustments within their component parts and with the environment.

- Systems use feedback both internally and externally. This is its mechanism for change.

- Systems are built on structures that provide the method for component interaction. This structure explains the operation of the system.

(von Bertalanffy, 1969)

lucky enough to sustain only a good scare. We might call this occurrence an event (or perhaps a low-consequence event). In contrast, if your car slides into a lane of oncoming traffic traveling at relatively high speeds, the consequences could be much more devastating: the state police may be called to respond to an accident and you could end up in the hospital, or worse.

System Events versus System Accidents

Any high-hazard operations can experience unplanned occurrences. In this guide, we use the following terms to denote the types of failures that can occur within a system:

- A *system event* is any unplanned, unforeseen occurrence that results from failure of the system, but does not result in catastrophic consequences (i.e., death, dose, dollars, delays, or one of the other "D" words). A system event may or may not disrupt the system operations. In fact, it may have virtually no actual consequences. Regardless of the level of consequence, a system event is always significant because it tells us that the system is not working as planned. A system event might be a precursor to a more consequential event or, under a different set of circumstances, might have resulted in the Big One. For example, in late August 2007, six cruise missiles, each loaded with a variable yield nuclear warhead, were mistakenly loaded on a United States Air Force B-52H heavy bomber at Minot Air Force Base and transported to Barksdale Air Force Base (Defense Science Board Permanent Task Force on Nuclear Weapons Surety, 2008). Although those directly affected by the event would argue, no severe

Chapter 1 | **13**

consequences occurred. The investigation, however, highlighted many organizational problems—some of which had their roots as far back as the fall of the Berlin Wall in the late 1980s. If left unchecked, these organizational failures could result in major consequences. Fortunately, information from the low-consequence system event has provided valuable insight into weaknesses within the system that can help the Air Force rectify ongoing problems.

- A *system accident* (also called an *organizational* or *normal accident*) may result from an unexpected single event that penetrates all existing system barriers or from the unanticipated interaction of multiple events. Either way, a system accident has serious consequences and causes total system disruption.

In a high-hazard operation, system events may occur occasionally, but a system accident is a rarity. An HRO strives to make system events rare and system accidents nonexistent.

System Accidents versus Individual Accidents
An important distinction must be made between a system accident, as described above, and what we will refer to in this guide as an *individual* accident. All accidents involve both an *agent* and a *victim*. The agent is the person, persons, or organization responsible for causing the accident, whereas the victim is the person, persons, or other entity that suffers the consequences of the accident. In an individual accident, the same person or group is both the agent and the victim. The car accident described earlier is an example of an individual accident.

System Events Spell Impending Disaster

The only things separating a system accident from a system event are the unrecoverable consequences. Both indicate a breakdown of the system, vital to the survivability of the company.

Don't wait for the Big One. Investigate significant information-rich system events—that is, low-consequence events that can tell you a lot about how the system is performing—to determine organizational weaknesses before they end in tragedy.

System Accidents Yield Disaster

The D-words are often used to describe the consequences of a system accident: death, dismemberment, damage, dose (radiation or chemical), dollars, days of lost production, discharges, delays, disruptions, discredit, disgrace, disaffected customers, departures of good employees, distraction of management focus, and demolition of assets.

(Corcoran, 2007b)

Safety Basis and Safe Operations

Organizations that deal with nuclear processes are familiar with the term *safety basis*, which is used by the U.S. Department of Energy (DOE) to indicate the level of rigor required by a nuclear facility to ensure safe operations and activities. The intent of a safety basis is to identify and document a comprehensive set of controls—administrative, technical and personnel—to establish a safety envelope within which operations can be safely carried out. The concept can also be applied to non-nuclear industries. For example, organizations that deal with chemical hazards must implement and document processes to prevent or mitigate impacts to on- and off-site populations from chemical-related accidents. These processes can be thought of as chemical safety basis.

It is important to understand and implement the requirements of the safety basis that applies to your industry; it is equally important not to be lulled into thinking that simply meeting these requirements is enough.

In contrast, a system accident can have devastating effects on populations, assets, and environments that were not involved in the circumstances or events leading to the accident. For example, the 1986 nuclear accident at Chernobyl was a system accident that resulted in deaths to emergency responders and negative health, socioeconomic, and environmental impacts to surrounding populations who had no involvement in the cause of the accident. Other examples of system accidents include the 2005 explosion at the BP Texas City refinery, the 1986 Challenger and 2003 Columbia space shuttle accidents, the Exxon Valdez oil spill in 1989, the 1979 nuclear accident at Three Mile Island, and the 1984 industrial disaster at the Union Carbide plant in Bhopal, India. In each case, uninvolved populations were affected and the results were disastrous in terms of human health and socioeconomic impacts.

Figure 1-1 illustrates the difference between individual and system accidents:

- In a system accident, the agent (typically, represented as human error) threatens the safety of the operation. This could lead to consequences which affect uninvolved victims within the organization, the local community, and the physical or socioeconomic environment. To prevent these consequences, the *hazard* (i.e., the operation or its hazardous component) must be protected from the *threat* (the agent, commonly human error or poor system design) through the use of a system.

- In an individual accident, the conditions of the workplace (i.e., the hazard) are a threat to the employee or other nearby persons (i.e.,

Chapter 1 | **15**

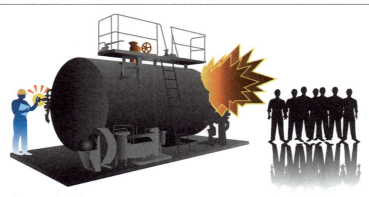

System Accident
In a system accident, individual errors threaten the safety of the operation (hazard) which could have a consequential impact on the local community, environment etc. (meltdown of a nuclear reactor, dispersal of hazardous chemicals, etc.), thus the hazard must be protected from human error through the use of a system.

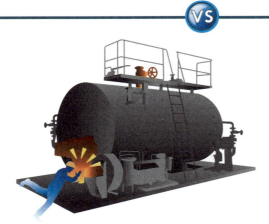

Individual Accident
In an individual accident, the conditions of the workplace (plant) are a threat to the employee, thus the employee must be protected from the plant. The hazards associated with individual accidents are typically addressed through industrial safety programs.

Figure 1-1. System versus Individual Accidents

the victim or victims), thus the employee must be protected from the hazard. The consequence associated with individual accidents is usually physical harm to the employee; prevention of this consequence is addressed through industrial safety programs.

Too frequently, the only barrier between a system event and a system accident is luck. In other words, many system events could become system accidents if the circumstances were slightly different—if, for example, the ambient air temperature had been only a few degrees higher or if there had been a car full of kids coming the other way when we hit the ice. Luck is not dependable, as any gambler knows. Nobody wants to gamble with a high-hazard operation; the stakes are simply too high. Instead, an HRO must focus its attention on seemingly small, unexpected system events to help diagnose and correct the underlying systemic problems before they escalate and result in system accidents with major consequences.

Lower the Threshold Of Concern

A system accident can occur despite numerous controls within the system. Thus, it is critical to take seriously any event that implicates problems with system integrity. Such an event should generate as much concern as if a catastrophic accident had occurred.

High-Hazard Operations: The Risk Factor

We've seen that the results of system accidents can be catastrophic, both for an organization and for the greater community. High-hazard operations face the highest possible consequences because of the nature of the materials and processes they use. It is because of these potentially serious consequences that HROs employ a systems approach to reduce the vulnerability to human error. However, the interacting, interrelated group of components that makes a system robust also introduces its own set of challenges. Hence the need to use a structured approach like that provided by Deming's Theory of Profound Knowledge (1994), which will be introduced later.

Is the risk—that is, the consequences compounded by the probability—of a system accident greater for high-hazard organizations than for other types of organizations? To explore the answer to this question, we must better understand some of the negative characteristics of systems that can lead to system accidents. When observed, these characteristics should serve as warning signals for an organization and spur them to greater efforts.

Charles Perrow (1999), a researcher who became very interested in how high-hazard organizations function after the 1979 accident at Three Mile Island, believes that system accidents are inevitable, albeit rare, in the complex systems that typify high-hazard technologies. In fact, he calls system accidents *normal accidents* because he believes they are bound to occur in the normal course of operations. Thus, an organization dealing with hazardous materials or processes that operates normally is doomed to experience a system (or normal) accident.

Perrow (1999) came to this conclusion because of his belief that high-hazard operations, particularly those involving nuclear technologies, have two characteristics that make them more prone to system accidents. He called these characteristics *complex interactivity* and *tight coupling*.

Complex Interactions Increase the Likelihood of Unexpected Events

As noted earlier, interactions among components of a system are inevitable because the components are interdependent. In many systems, such interactions are expected and familiar, and the sequence of events is visible. These types of interactions are labeled linear interactions. In a linear interaction, when an unplanned sequence occurs, the employees can immediately locate and remedy the problem. For example, in an automobile assembly line, the employees can visibly see when there is a holdup.

Some high-hazard operations, however, can be characterized by complex interactions. Many of these interactions are either not visible or not immediately comprehensible by those having to make time-critical operational decisions. In a nuclear reactor, for example, the critical components must be located in close proximity or within the sealed reactor vessel. As a result, they are not visible and the operators must rely on numerous (and fallible) warning devices. According to Perrow (1999), organizations and systems with high degrees of interactive complexity are likely to experience unexpected and often baffling interactions among components, interactions that designers may not have anticipated and operators cannot recognize within the required reaction time. Consequently, they are highly vulnerable to common-mode failures. Although designers and operators attempt to anticipate all likely potential problems, it is typically an unlikely failure—whether bizarre or commonplace—that initiates a system accident.

Tight Coupling Increases the Likelihood That Events Will Escalate

System coupling refers to the degree to which subsystems and units are linked and interdependent. In a loosely coupled system, the operations and processes may progress independently. Delays can be tolerated: unfinished products can sit for periods without damage, processes can be repeated, if necessary, and the system can be placed in standby mode. Ample time is available to improvise, when needed.

Common-mode Failure
This type of failure occurs when a single event causes multiple systems to fail. For example, if all of the pumps for a fire sprinkler system are located in one room and the room becomes too hot for the pumps to operate, they will all fail at essentially the same time from a common cause (the high temperature).

(Wikipedia, 2007)

Tightly-coupled systems have more time-dependent processes, therefore planned and unplanned interactions occur quickly. In tightly-coupled systems, the sequence and coordinated activities needed to produce a product are invariant (there is only one way to make the product, and the process must proceed in an established sequence). Tightly-coupled systems have little slack—quantities used in production must be precise, and the process must be done correctly or not at all. In tightly-coupled systems, safety devices, redundancies, and buffers between parts and the production process are limited to those that were planned and designed into the system. If the tightly-coupled systems interact more quickly than the operators can respond, an event can escalate into a full-blown system accident before the operator can react.

Organizations can exhibit interactive complexity, but can be either tightly- or loosely-coupled. For example, a large university has complex interactions but loose coupling, whereas a nuclear power plant is both interactively complex and tightly-coupled. Although interactive complexity increases the likelihood of dangerous incidents, it is tight coupling that will cause the incidents to escalate to a full-blown system accident with major consequences.

Managing Human Error: The Pitfalls of Redundancy

Nearly all investigations into system accidents discover that human error was a major contributor to the accident. In fact, as shown in Figure 1-1, it is typically the threat of human error that makes the hazard—whether mechanical, chemical, biological, or nuclear—vulnerable. It is human nature to err. According to recent research, an

---

Redundancy

The principle of redundancy states that, when events of failure of a component are statistically independent, the probabilities of their joint occurrence multiply. Thus, for instance, if the probability of failure of a component of a system is 1 in 1000 per year, the probability of the joint failure of two of them is 1 in 1 million per year, provided that the two events are statistically independent. This principle favors the strategy of the redundancy of components.

A prime example of redundancy with isolation is a nuclear power plant. The new advanced boiling water reactor has three divisions of emergency core cooling systems, each with its own generators and pumps and each isolated from the others. The new European pressurized reactor has two containment buildings, one inside the other. However, even here it is not impossible for a common-mode failure to occur (for example, caused by a highly-unlikely Richter 10 earthquake).

(Wikipedia, 2007)

individual is expected to make four to five errors an hour, on average (INPO, 2006).

High-hazard operations attempt to minimize vulnerability from human fallibility by using redundant systems, processes, and employees. Redundancy helps achieve reliability through duplication and overlap of effort. The key is not simply to achieve redundancy, but to achieve *independent redundancy* (Figure 1-2). Independent barriers or defenses accommodate human fallibility while maintaining the safety envelope that protects the hazardous operation. For example, if your job is to turn off steam valves before opening the steam line to perform work, you may want to have someone check that the valve is indeed closed before you begin work. The best approach is to have the person check independently to ensure the valve is closed. Of course, you could save time by having the verifier accompany you and watch as you close the valve; however, it is important to note that this is not independent verification. The danger is that if the verifier is not directly responsible, she may assume you are shutting the line off even if the valve isn't completely closed.

There is a negative side to redundancy, however, as Charles Perrow (1999) warns. Redundancy can increase the likelihood, although not the escalation, of unexpected system events for three reasons:

The key is not simply to achieve redundancy, but to achieve independent redundancy.

- First, although redundant backups are supposed to be independent, they could increase the interactive complexity of highly technical operations and lead to unanticipated common-mode failures.

- Second, adding redundancy could make the system more opaque, which could make failures of individual components or employees less obvious, since overlap of backup devices or backup personnel compensates for any such failure.

- Third, although redundancy makes the system appear safer, operators may take advantage of this perceived security to push the system to higher levels of performance.

The presence of sophisticated system or component redundancy, also called defenses-in-depth redundancy, has changed the character of industrial accidents more than any other factor, making modern technological systems largely immune to isolated failures. Yet, according to Perrow's concept of normal accidents, **redundant barriers may also be the single feature most responsible for the emergence of system accidents because they tend to increase interactive complexity, obscure failures that have no immediate consequences, and breed complacency, which results in unsafe practices (Perrow, 1999).**

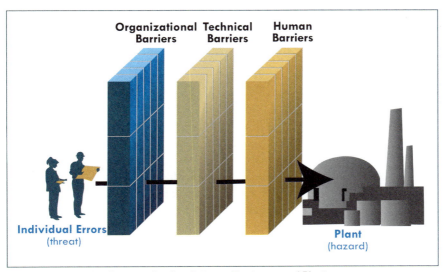

Figure 1-2. Redundant Systems: Barriers Between Employees and Plant

High Reliability Operations • A Practical Guide to Avoid the System Accident

Are High-hazard Operations More Prone to System Accidents?

Perrow (1999) claims that high-hazard operations that operate normally will inevitably lead to system accidents. Is this true of your operation? All of us would like to think that because of the built-in safeguards and operational procedures associated with our high-hazard facilities, an extraordinary number of things must go wrong for a catastrophe to occur, and yet catastrophic system accidents such as the Three Mile Island nuclear reactor accident do continue to occur. Why? Is our safety success our worst enemy?

Our contention is that the success of the systems we put in place to prevent the catastrophic event often results in complacency. Daily operations are characterized by unexpected events and human error; the danger of complacency is that it leads an organization to self-satisfaction, which places focus on strengths rather than weaknesses and encourages managers and employees to "let down their guard."

How does your organization operate? Are you confident your operations are safe or are you simply crossing your fingers? Does your organization operate as an HRO? Anything you can do to make your operations safer, while still ensuring that your products and services remain dependable and of high quality, deserves judicious consideration. Remaining vigilant to system weaknesses and learning from those weaknesses is critical to ensure high reliability operations. But how does an organization guard against the natural tendency towards the normal organization introduced by Perrow (1999)?

A Practical Systems Approach to High Reliability: Four Guiding Practices

As managers and engineers who work in an organization characterized by high-hazard operations, we asked ourselves this very question. To answer it, we studied existing literature about HROs, searching for information that would help transform our operations. Our goal was to discover not just what approaches and tools to use to become an HRO, but why we should use them. Toward this end, we studied the Normal Accident Theory of Perrow (1999) to understand the pitfalls of most high-hazard operations. We read books and articles by various researchers interested in High Reliability Theory, system accidents, and safety culture (Sagan, 1993; Weick and Sutcliffe, 2001; Reason, 1990, 1997, 1998; Dekker, 2006; Hopkins, 2002, 2006a, 2006b, 2007; Schein, 1992, 1999, 2004) to help us understand the characteristics and practices of HROs.

Like others before us (Marais et al., 2004) we began to examine how a top-down systems approach could provide the platform we need for practical implementation. We became interested in the *mindful approach* that HROs should use to manage unexpected events, as promulgated by Weick and Sutcliffe (2001). From this it was evident that a systems approach was required to reduce the vulnerabilities resulting from our human errors and systems design. Hence we needed a systematic and robust way of managing the HRO system. We also wanted to go beyond simply propagating a list of HRO heuristics based on observations of high-hazard operations with good track records. We wanted to know the why behind the what, so that an organization could understand how to adapt HRO practices to their own business.

Our search for a systematic way to manage the HRO system led us to W.E. Deming's Theory of Profound Knowledge (1994), which served as an umbrella under which we could assimilate our own practical experience as well as information gleaned from other theories. Deming's theory, first published in 1994, is a synthesis of previous theories related to systems and statistical process control[2]. In its most basic form, it can be boiled down to four basic tenets, which Deming claims are interrelated and inseparable:

- **Knowledge of systems.** A system, says Deming, is a network of interdependent components working together to accomplish a specific aim. Systems must be managed; they tend to perpetuate their own goals and resist change. The greater the interdependence between components, the greater the need for communication and cooperation among these components and the greater the need for overall management. Failure of management to comprehend the interdependence between components can be the cause of loss. The efforts of the various divisions in a company, each given a job, are not additive but interdependent. Each component part is obligated to contribute its best to the system rather than maximize its own profit, and may even operate at a loss in order to optimize the entire system.

- **Knowledge of variation.** Everything in life is variable. This is particularly true when dealing with human systems. Organizations can deal with variability by first measuring it using tools such as statistics—numerical estimates based on a sample or samples—to predict outcomes. When dealing with processes, for example, statistics can be used to define process capability, thus making performance predictable. Based on comparing predictions versus performance, variation can be controlled. This principle applies to people and systems as well as processes. Knowledge about the different sources of uncertainty should be used to refine the system or process being implemented (i.e., to reduce variability). Measurement is an iterative process; it is not to be performed just once.

- **Knowledge of psychology.** A leader of transformation must learn and understand the psychology of individuals, the psychology of a group (commonly called the culture of the organization), and the psychology of change. Psychology helps managers understand people; the interaction between people and systems; the interaction between customer and supplier; and the interaction between managers, employees, and any system of management.

- **Knowledge of knowledge.** Management in any form is prediction. Managers predict future outcome, with the risk of being wrong, based on observations of the past. Rational prediction builds knowledge through the systematic revision and extension of theoretical principles; such revision is based on a comparison of prediction and observation. Feedback helps validate, improve, or invalidate the theory. Without theory, there is no learning. It is only in a state of statistical control that statistical theory provides, with a high degree of belief, prediction of performance in the immediate future. Information, no matter how complete and immediate, is not knowledge. Knowledge has temporal spread and develops from the testing of theory. Without a theory against which to test the information, there is no way to use information received at a specific point in time (Deming, 1994).

The simplicity, and perhaps also the difficulty, of implementing Deming's theory lies with the integration of these four principles. Many organizations implement these elements individually to some degree but fail to comprehend the synergy among them and the significance of the continuous cycle they form. This cycle is illustrated in Figure 1-3. The interaction among Deming's basic tenets—the knowledge of systems, variability, psychology, and knowledge—may occur in any order or direction.

We began to compare the information we obtained about high-hazard operations and HROs from our literature review and our own experience against the system structure provided by Deming's theory. What we discovered surprised us—Deming's Theory of Profound Knowledge provided a robust framework that allowed us to further develop key HRO practices for a broad range of organizations. In essence, Deming's theory could explain why HROs could work, not just describe their outward trappings. Using this framework and drawing on the theories of other researchers, validated from our own experience, we developed four HRO practices that can be applied to almost any industry. We describe these practices, which are overlain on Deming's Theory of Profound Knowledge in Figure 1-3, as follows:

- Manage the system, not the parts

- Reduce system variability

- Foster a strong culture of reliability

- Learn and adapt as an organization

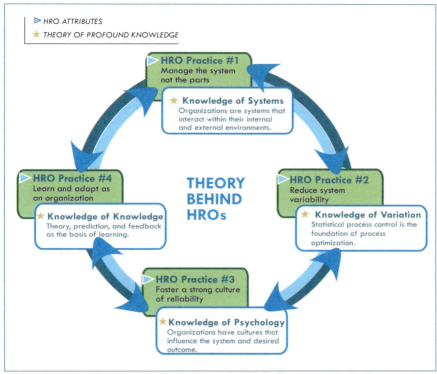

Figure 1-3. The Four HRO Practices and Their Relationship to the Theory of Profound Knowledge (Deming, 1994)

In a healthy HRO, these practices will be internalized to the degree that they inform all major management decisions. As such, they are integral to the approaches and tools we present in this guide.

Manage the System, Not the Parts

This practice is related to Deming's knowledge of systems (Figure 1-3) and focuses on, and must be implemented by, managers. Without management buy-in and commitment there is no HRO. Deming was right on mark when he stated that a system, which represents a network of interdependent components working together to accomplish a specific aim, must be managed. Thus, although systems provide powerful defenses to protect against catastrophic accidents, they also present a new set of challenges to managers. The organizational interdependence exhibited by systems results in a tendency toward self perpetuation of goals and resistance to change. As Deming stated, the greater the interdependence between components, the greater the need for communications and management.

Deming also indicated that system performance issues often have their genesis in the design and management of the system. System failures are rooted in the complex interactions between system components and human failures; as the complexity of such interactions increases, accidents caused by dysfunctional component interactions are more likely. Thus, managers who implement a system approach to reduce the vulnerability of the system to human error must be careful that the system interactions don't introduce new failure mechanisms with unforeseen consequences. Not only must managers oversee the development and deployment of the system, they must have a relentless drive to obtain accurate, timely, and continuous feedback on its overall health. Managers must be courageous enough to persevere even when initiatives are difficult to implement and measure, and must communicate their commitment to safety and reliability not only through their talk but also through their actions. That is, the manager must foster an organizational culture that expects and acts upon open and honest communication from the workforce, and thus encourages continuous organizational learning and adapting.

Reduce System Variability

To function as an HRO, an organization must deploy a robust HRO system, evaluate the performance of the system, and continuously reduce performance variability to decrease the likelihood of unexpected system events. This directly relates to Deming's knowledge of variation (Figure 1-3). Although Deming focuses on the use of statistics to measure and reduce variation, each organization must determine the type of evaluation system most appropriate for its operations.

In this guide, we introduce a six-step HRO process we call the Break-the-Chain Framework. Within this HRO framework, variability is reduced by minimizing hazards, reducing the negative influences of complex interactivity and tight coupling, minimizing human error, and employing redundant independent barriers as backup measures in case other actions fail.

Feedback, corrective actions, and organizational learning are key to reducing variation in the Break-the-Chain Framework. To ensure proper feedback, managers must clarify what they want reported and choose monitoring metrics wisely. Employees must understand what is considered a deviation from the norm if they are expected to spot such deviations early and take corrective action.

Foster a Strong Culture of Reliability

As no system works unless it is used, managers should encourage employees to fully implement, believe, and police the use of the HRO system. As no system is perfect, managers should encourage employees to challenge the system and thus identify system shortcomings before they result in unanticipated events (Deming's knowledge

HRO Management Must Be Transparent

"Transparency in leadership means not only stating the goals but demonstrating adherence to those espoused values through everyday personal examples. It also requires that there are mechanisms in place to provide feedback about goal attainment in a way that allows everyone to see the progress of the organization."

(Corcoran, 2007a).

of psychology, Figure 1-3). To encourage these behaviors requires that managers learn and understand the psychology of individuals, groups, and change so that they better understand people, the interaction between people and circumstances, and the interactions among managers, employees, and any system of management. This equates to understanding the culture of the organization. We use the term *culture of reliability* in this guide to indicate an organizational culture that focuses not only on safety, but on consistent, dependable, and excellent products and services. A culture of reliability, according to our definition, encompasses three concepts:

- Employees who are trained, empowered, and expected to make conservative decisions on the shop floor.

- Employees who retain their proficiency through continual hands-on work.

- An organization (managers and employees) that transparently demonstrates its culture of reliability by walking the talk, and challenging and acting to improve unsafe conditions to protect against the system accident.

To have a strong culture of reliability, the managers of an HRO need to be learners and strategists; they must never be satisfied with the status quo, and must constantly push for improvement within the context of the organization's strategic plan and objectives. Managers must constantly reinforce the desired cultural traits through words, actions, and decisions.

Learn and Adapt as an Organization

As stated earlier, HROs cannot measure their success solely in terms of safety statistics. HROs must be learning organizations that strive for excellence through continuous organizational renewal (Deming's knowledge of knowledge, Figure 1-3). Because safety is a core value for an HRO, the aim is to gather as much relevant information as possible and turn it into knowledge that can be applied to the organization. The continuous flow of cross-functional information is essential to learning. To support this need for information, HROs need an effective mechanism of reporting that includes feedback mechanisms.

Deming states that management, in any form, is prediction. Unfortunately, the cost of uncertainty in prediction is great for a high-hazard operation. The most effective measure of the degree of uncertainty in high-hazard operations is to evaluate the gaps between work-as-imagined (i.e., the work processes as dictated by the HRO system and desired by management) and work-as-done by the employee. Deming (1994) introduced a cycle of planning, doing, checking, and acting (PDCA) as a methodology to build knowledge through systematic revision and extension of theoretical principles. Using this as a basis, we suggest a five-tiered approach to organizational learning that provides feedback from start-up processes, daily supervisor-employee interactions, tracking and trending of data, Causal Factors Analysis, and organization/external lessons. When a deviation from the norm is observed, feedback about the deviation is compared against the Break-the-Chain Framework in a backward-stepping fashion to highlight weak points in the system. These various levels of feedback and learning allow us to gain a true understanding of the underlying causes of the deviation—which frequently reflect poor system design or problems at the organizational culture level—and, if necessary, to better refine the system and manage the culture to achieve specific goals.

The Alternative To High Reliability Operations —The System Accident:

- 1906 Courrières, France Mine Disaster – 1099 killed

- 1921 Oppau, Germany Fertilizer Plant Explosion – 600 killed

- 1944 Port of Chicago Naval Magazine Explosion – 320 killed

- 1932-1968 Minamata Japan Mercury Poisoning – 3000 deformities

- 1965 Little Rock Titan Missile Fire – 53 killed

- 1976 Seveso Italy Dioxin Release – 70,000 animals slaughtered

- 1989, 1999, and 2000 Phillips Explosions & Fires – 26 killed, 389 injured

- 1993 Kadar Toy Factory Fire Thailand – 188 killed

- 2001 China Mine Accident – 81 killed

- 2005 Ghotki, Pakistan Train Accident – 127 killed

The cost to implement continuous learning within an organization is high, and the competition for resources is real in every organization. An HRO must ensure that commitment, systems, and resources are in place that will allow it to doubt, challenge, learn, and adapt as an organization through the trials of daily operations.

The HRO Journey: What You Should Know Before You Go

An organization can be healthy and profitable, and can offer a safe work environment even though it is not an HRO. Before embarking on the HRO journey, senior management should ensure that the organization's managers share both the desire and commitment to become an HRO. A journey can be a pleasurable experience or a miasma of unfortunate events; an organization's journey toward HRO status is no different, regardless of whether the final destination is reached. Some organizations will never make it to the final destination, and others may be disappointed once they arrive. The journey may offer more opportunity for learning and growth than the destination itself.

Each organization's journey to become an HRO will be different. Most will be difficult, as organizational change is not easy. Commitment from senior management, coupled with a strong desire to learn a new way of doing business, the patience to see it through, and the willingness to allocate necessary resources are all necessary. Without such commitment and support, the success of the journey is questionable.

It may be true, as Perrow (1999) claims, that no high-technology, high-hazard operation can ever be completely safe and reliable. System accidents may be inevitable, given enough time.

Our position, however, is that awareness of this possibility is the first step in making your operations safer. Daily vigilance and chronic unease are critical for safety.

The following chapter presents information to help you better understand the four HRO practices, which embody the major characteristics of an HRO and thus represent the end state of the HRO journey. We recommend that you use this chapter to help you determine if the HRO journey is appropriate and feasible for your organization. If you decide to embark on the journey, Chapter 3 will guide you through the strategic planning process needed to become an HRO.

Chapters 4 through 7, which represent the implementing and sustaining phase of the HRO journey, focus on tools that will help you nourish and maintain high reliability operations. Chapter 8 provides a summary of the highlights presented in this guide and provides you with a set of pointers to help you as a manager of an HRO.

The organization of this guide, along with the questions each chapter answers is provided in the road map presented in Figure 1-4. This road map to becoming an HRO provides a framework for reading and understanding this text.

Sustaining the HRO practices over time is perhaps the most difficult aspect of the HRO journey, and reflects our belief that the journey never really ends. Those of us who work with and manage high-hazard operations can never afford to relax our efforts to improve the safety and reliability of our organizations. We must always expect the unexpected.

Figure 1-4. Roadmap to High Reliability Operations

Understanding	Planning		Implementing
CHAPTER 1 Knowing what it means to be an HRO	**CHAPTER 2** Knowing where you are headed (HRO Practice 1 Manage the System, not the Parts)	**CHAPTER 3** Transforming your organization to an HRO (HRO Practice 1 Manage the System, not the Parts)	**CHAPTER 4** Breaking the chain between threat and hazard (HRO Practice 2 Reduce System Variability)
• What is an HRO? • My high-hazard operation has an excellent safety record—does that mean it is an HRO? • Why should my organization strive to become an HRO? • What is a system accident and how does it differ from other types of accidental events I am trying to prevent? • Is my high-hazard organization more prone to system accidents than other operations? • Why is a systems approach necessary to prevent the accident my organization fears most? • What are four organizational practices that will enable my organization to nourish and support high reliability operations?	• What does it mean to manage the system? • What does it take to reduce system variability? • What will it take to help my organization foster a culture of reliability? • What does it mean to be a learning organization and how can I, as a manager, encourage this trait? • What will it take to assimilate the four HRO practices into my organization's operations?	• How does my organization develop a strategy for becoming an HRO? • What are the seven elements used to drive a systems approach to transformation? • How are the four HRO practices used to inform strategy development? • How does my organization develop objectives and indicators? • How does my organization measure the effectiveness of the transformation process?	• What are the six common pitfalls that an HRO must avoid? • What does it mean to break the chain from threat to hazard? • How does the Break-the-Chain Framework relate to the four HRO practices? • What are the six steps of the Break-the-Chain Framework? • How can my organization evaluate its safety system and adjust its processes?

Figure 1-4. Roadmap to High Reliability Operations

Implementing	Sustaining		
CHAPTER 5 Fostering a culture of reliability (HRO Practice 3 Foster a Strong Culture of Reliability)	**CHAPTER 6** Learning and adapting as an organization (HRO Practice 4 Learn & Adapt as an Organization)	**CHAPTER 7** Evaluating your organization's culture of reliability as a measure of effectiveness of HRO practices	**CHAPTER 8** Wrapping it up
• Why is organizational culture important to an HRO? • What is the difference between a safety culture and a culture of reliability? • Why does my HRO organization need to foster a culture of reliability? • How do I, as a manager, foster a culture of reliability?	• As a manager, how do I generate decision-making information? • What sort of feedback is associated with each of the five tiers of generating organizational learning? • How do I manage to ensure that feedback about the safety system is appropriately interpreted and integrated into day-to-day operations? • How do I use feedback to refine the HRO safety system?	• How do I characterize my organization's culture of reliability? • How can I use this characterization to evaluate my organization's culture of reliability? • What does the health of my organization's culture of reliability tell me about the effectiveness of my HRO? • If I discover indications of an unhealthy culture, how can I go about improving it?	• How does Deming's Theory of Profound Knowledge support and inform the four HRO practices? • Are the four HRO practices distinct or interrelated? • How does an organization begin the HRO transformation process? • How does an organization sustain high reliability operations? • What "pearls of wisdom" can I take away from this guide to help me in my day-to-day management of an HRO?

Chapter 2

Chapter 2

Knowing Where You Are Headed: How to Manage the System

This chapter answers the following questions:

- What does it mean to manage the system?

- What does it take to reduce system variability?

- What will it take to help my organization foster a culture of reliability?

- What does it mean to be a learning organization and how can I, as a manager, encourage this trait?

- What will it take to assimilate the four HRO practices into my organization's operations?

The four guiding practices of an HRO, as presented in Chapter 1, create a synergy that helps sustain safe, reliable operations. If your organization decides to undertake the HRO journey, your aim, as a manager, should be to assimilate these practices into your daily operations.

This chapter focuses on HRO Practice 1, Manage the System, Not the Parts. This practice frames the responsibilities and expectations of managers with respect to the other three HRO practices (which are discussed in more detail in Chapters 4 through 6). It is through HRO Practice 1 that you, as a manager, will drive the development and the integration of the other three HRO practices to sustain safe, reliable operations. In addition to helping you and your organization make an

---

The Four HRO Practices

1 Manage the system, not the parts

2 Reduce system variability

3 Foster a strong culture of reliability

4 Learn and adapt as an organization

HRO Practice 1: Manage The System, Not The Parts

This practice requires managers to take actions that:

- Ensure the safety system selected provides safety

- Manage the safety system to reduce variability

- Foster a culture of reliability

- Model organizational learning

informed decision about undertaking the HRO journey, knowledge of HRO Practice 1 will help you visualize the final destination so that you can devise strategies to get there. Thus, we introduce all four HRO practices in this chapter with the intent of showing the leadership attitudes and actions necessary to implement these practices.

Keep in mind that the realization of the HRO ideal is ephemeral, at best. The daily struggle to be an HRO will continue long after your organization has met all its strategic targets, and will require constant review and expansion of these four HRO practices into every facet of daily operations. Like all organizations striving for greatness, an HRO can never maintain steady state; consequently, it is either declining toward a lower energy state or revving up to a higher energy state. Your job as a manager is to measure and monitor the system to catch decline, then set the organization on a corrective path to get back into equilibrium or to strive for a higher level of reliability.

Manage the System, Not the Parts

As Deming (1994) points out, a system must be managed; our contention is that a healthy organizational system is managed consciously from the top down. As a manager, you are responsible for guiding your operation or organization to the desired destination. To do this, you must have a shared vision and a plan for attaining that vision. In Chapter 3, we describe how you can achieve this by implementing a transformation strategy whose components are designed to close the gap between current operational practices and the desired HRO practices.

The focus of HRO Practice 1 is to explain and clarify what your organizational expectations should be, both during and after the transformation to an HRO. As such, HRO Practice 1 provides the motivation and framework for implementing the other three HRO practices introduced in this text. HRO Practice 1 demands that you maintain a systems perspective and strive relentlessly to obtain accurate, timely, and continuous feedback about the health of the organizational system.

To ensure the HRO system is aligned with organizational priorities, you must clearly articulate operational goals and plans in an open and transparent manner.[3] As a manager, you must verify that the HRO system adopted—whether it is the Break-the-Chain Framework described in this guide or another safety system[4]—actually provides the level of safety required to prevent the feared catastrophic event (HRO Practice 2). This requires careful design, adaptation, and on-the-ground implementation—the HRO safety system will not work if it is viewed simply as a paperwork exercise to cover your tail. Because catastrophic events are rare, you must continually and forcefully drive the development, implementation, and refinement of the HRO systems in the face of complacency about such events. Also, you must convince employees to buy into the system, despite its warts (and no system is perfect). This can be done through a process of intense training that encourages employees to challenge and strengthen the system, and to police it in an attempt to guard against those who vary from its requirements. You must foster a culture of reliability (HRO Practice 3) in which all employees insist that operations be performed in a safe manner. Key to this process is continuous

Ownership

"A person doing a job—any job—must feel that he owns it and that he will remain on that job indefinitely. Lack of commitment to the present job will be perceived by those who work for him, and they will also tend not to care. If he feels he owns his job and acts accordingly, he need not worry about his next job."

(Rickover)

Safety Culture

A safety culture is an organization's values and behaviors, modeled by its leaders, and internalized by its members, that serve to make safe performance of work the overriding priority to protect the public, employees, and the environment.

(Adapted from INPO, 2004)

Culture of Reliability

We use the term culture of reliability in this guide to denote a positive safety culture characterized by "communications founded on mutual trust, by shared perceptions of the importance of safety, and by confidence in the efficacy of preventive measures."

(ACSNI, 1993)

Positive Control

What happens is what we intended to happen and that is all that happens

(INPO, 2006, p.51)

Facing The Facts

"Another principle for managing a successful program is to resist the natural human inclination to hope things will work out, despite evidence or doubt to the contrary. It is not easy to admit that what you thought was correct did not turn out that way. If conditions require it, one must face the facts and brutally make needed changes despite considerable costs and schedule delays. The man in charge must personally set the example in this area."

(Rickover)

organizational learning to adapt to daily challenges (HRO Practice 4).

Throughout this effort, you must walk the talk. **No matter what level of the organization you manage, you must continually demonstrate the importance of system safety and reliability, every day through every action you take.** Perceived insincerity will be reflected in an unhealthy safety culture that will not only undermine HRO programs, but also the industrial safety programs put in place to reduce individual accidents.

Ensure the Safety System Selected Provides Safety

If you, as a manager, plan to rely on an HRO system to prevent a catastrophic accident, you must ensure the selected safety system does provide the requisite level of protection. High-hazard operations are a good example of Deming's claim that system performance issues often begin with the design of the system, as they require a level of physical safety that must be built into the system. No amount of paperwork will prevent a catastrophic accident.

To ensure the proper safety system is selected, you must have an in-depth understanding of the technical aspects of the business you manage. This knowledge is needed to ensure the safety system and controls will protect the specific hazard (whether that is a plant that could explode, an airplane or space shuttle that could crash, or a biological or radiological agent that could be released into the environment) from the agent or threat (typically, human error but could also originate from poor system design). You must verify—not assume, hope, or imagine—that the system provides the required level of safety and nothing more. This is important: if additional nonessential system safety requirements are added to the system, eventually the focus on the true hazards will be diluted.

Along with a technical understanding of the business, you must also understand the precepts of high reliability operations and the warning signs of pending system accidents in order to understand what you are trying to avoid. You must struggle to understand what a culture of reliability is, and become comfortable with methods to evaluate the culture of your organization. This will help you evaluate the effectiveness of the HRO programs you are trying to implement.

Manage the Safety System to Reduce Variability

With the proper safety system selected, the next challenge for you is to develop and deploy that system throughout the operation or organization. It is important that you not lose sight of the goal during this process. Managers often feel the pressure to reduce the number of lost-time or recordable injuries and achieve enviable lost-time rates. Remember, however, that the HRO system is meant to prevent a system accident, which can potentially kill or injure hundreds of people, not to lower the number of individual accidents. If you lose sight of this goal, you may end up redirecting the priorities of your operation and thus fail in reaching your goal of becoming an HRO.

With the above in mind, you must stress the need to minimize the consequences associated with the hazards of your operation by publishing and continuously reminding your employees of the hazards. Every action you take should be focused on preventing the consequential system

Priorities

"If you are to manage your job, you must set priorities. Too many people let the job set the priorities. You must apply self-discipline to ensure your energy is applied where it is most needed."

(Rickover)

Responsibility

"Along with ownership comes the need for full acceptance of full responsibility for the work. Shared responsibility means that no one is responsible. Unless one person who is truly responsible can be identified when something goes wrong, then no one has really been responsible."

(Rickover)

accident—at all costs and at all times. Be careful not to divert needed resources in an attempt to prevent less consequential events if such diversion of resources will reduce the effectiveness of the system with respect to the system accident. Keep in mind the proverb "Disaster strikes when you least expect it," and make sure that you and your employees are on guard at all times. This is not to say ignore industrial safety programs, but rather don't keep investing in those programs to the exclusion of the bigger consequence event. Balance is the key.

To prevent the system accident, you must ensure that your operation follows the established safety system, regardless of the impact it may have on production. Because it involves people, equipment, and processes, the safety system is dynamic and requires the continuous influx of resources and support infrastructure to maintain its viability. Only you, as the manager, can provide these key ingredients. You must ensure the right people are in the right job to preclude degradation of the safety within your operation.

Because no system is perfect and all systems are dynamic, you must continually evaluate the safety system against its design metrics in an effort to detect points where common-mode failures may occur. Variations within the established safety system must be noted and reduced, and the system must be continuously refined to optimize processes and remove no-value added requirements.

As mentioned in Chapter 1, we have developed an HRO safety system called the Break-the-Chain Framework. Although it was designed to prevent a catastrophic event, it can also be used in reverse as an investigative tool to systematically evaluate unexpected system events. This framework, described in detail in Chapter 4, incorporates the safety practices described above, as well as many aspects of the other three high-level HRO practices.

Foster a Culture of Reliability

To truly be effective, the HRO system must be used by all employees at all times. This requires a significant commitment and a large outlay of resources, which is borne partly by the customers of the business. As a manager, you are responsible for ensuring your employees are capable of, and empowered to make, conservative decisions regarding going outside of the adopted safety system. This requires providing them with the proper training, arming them with the proper tools, and providing them with support that allows them to effectively use their skills without being distracted by unnecessary side issues. But your role does not stop here. As a manager of a high-hazard operation, you must provide your employees with continuous hands-on experience to keep their skills sharp and their awareness keen. In this way, you will ensure they can make fact-based decisions if the need arises.

Chapter 5 provides an in-depth discussion of the practical steps needed to foster a culture of reliability. Keep in mind, however, that the HRO system you select will require continued scrutiny and refinement based on real-life use. You must instill a sense of trust among your employees that encourages them to openly identify, report, and share errors among the whole organization. Through your actions to resolve issues, you should support open communications and insist on a healthy questioning attitude among your employees and fellow managers. In short, you must develop a chronic unease about day-to-day

Know What Is Going On

"You must establish simple and direct means to find out what is going on in detail in the area of your responsibility. I require regular periodic reports directly to me from personnel throughout my program."

(Rickover)

Pay Attention To Detail

"A tendency among managers, particularly as they move to higher positions, is to think they no longer need to be concerned with details. If the boss is not concerned about details, his subordinates also will not consider them important."

(Rickover)

operations that is manifested in questioning, requires resolution, and results in the appropriate corrective action.

Model Organizational Learning

Because safety is never the only goal of an operation, you should expect daily struggles to deal with conflicts between performance and safety. You should address these struggles openly and take care to think through the entire life-cycle of a process before making a decision. It is critical that you, as a manager, demonstrate a genuine desire to know the health of the business and are courageous enough to address the issues, not just the symptoms. Consider employee performance as an indicator of the safety culture and take steps to manage the culture if it does not support the goal of the HRO. This requires you to use every available means to obtain feedback. You can obtain the most reliable feedback first hand by walking the shop floors and talking directly to employees. In Chapter 6, we present a five-tiered approach to improve organizational learning, which discusses various means of obtaining feedback. Tier 3 of this method focuses on an investigative process we call Causal Factors Analysis (CFA), which is the focus of the companion volume to this guide, *Causal Factors Analysis: An Approach to Organizational Learning* (Hartley et al., 2008). Integrating and interpreting the data from CFA and other sources is key to helping you evaluate the effectiveness of your HRO system. Using this information to continually refine your HRO system will ensure the viability of your operations.

Making the Practices Work: A Mindful Approach

HRO Practice 1 and the other three HRO practices it frames are not conceptually difficult; in fact, they may seem like common sense. The difficulty lies in understanding how they can be assimilated into your current organization in a way that is both sustainable and measurable. If you are successful at assimilating these practices, you should begin to see signs of what Weick and Suttcliffe (2001) describe as mindfulness. Knowledge of this concept will help you, as a manager, better understand how the four HRO practices contribute to and inform one another.

To sustain the four HRO practices within an organization requires its managers to be mindful about ongoing operations. In other words, you—as a manager—must be continually aware of the current state of affairs and attuned to possible changes that could signal potential trouble. In their book *Managing the Unexpected*, Weick and Sutcliffe (2001) provide insight into the importance of management behavior for high reliability operations. They claim that **high reliability operations can be sustained only if an organization actively anticipates and manages the unexpected.** This involves possessing an awareness that the unexpected can—and will—happen, as well as the presence of mind and in-place processes to contain unexpected events and prevent them from escalating. Such a state of readiness requires a state of mindfulness.

Mindfulness, according to Weick and Sutcliffe (2001), is what allows an HRO to be alert to the first sign of trouble. Such signals may be weak in comparison to the noise of everyday operations. The negative characteristics typically associated with high-hazard operations become more prevalent when an organization operates mindlessly—that is, when it understands neither itself nor its environment and is essentially preoccupied with upholding and updating the status quo. Awareness of possible dangers (i.e., chronic unease) and continual vigilance are key to achieving and maintaining high reliability operations. Weick and Sutcliffe claim that employees of HROs are able to recognize and cope with the unexpected because they collect multiple signals (Deming, 1994) from a variety of sources and assemble these signals to determine where aberrations from the planned HRO practices occur.[5] When these data are inconclusive, HRO employees assume that danger is imminent and act accordingly. In this way, awareness of the pitfalls described by Perrow's Normal Accident Theory (1999) can help operators of high-hazard operations to remain vigilant.

Five sustaining characteristics are required to maintain a mindful outlook; we believe these characteristics should be considered hallmarks of an HRO:

- Reluctance to simplify

- Preoccupation with failure

- Sensitivity to operations

- Commitment to resilience

- Deference to expertise

As shown in Figure 2-1, organizations that exhibit these characteristics encourage a process of questioning, reaffirmation or adaptation, and learning that results in mindfulness. This allows an organization to identify and address the minor symptoms of systemic illness before these symptoms result in a system accident with consequential results.

As the manager of an organization striving to implement the four HRO practices, you should

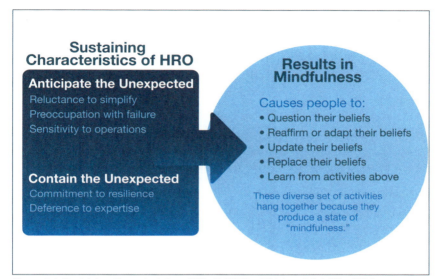

Figure 2-1. Sustaining Characteristics of Mindful HROs (Weick and Sutcliffe, 2001)

determine whether you and your employees operate in a mindful manner. To help you in this regard, Table 2-1 cross-walks the characteristics of mindfulness with the four HRO practices. In actuality, there are many additional parallels between the HRO practices and the characteristics of mindfulness—you may think of additional commonalities within your organization as you examine this table. Such overlap reflects how the practices themselves are intertwined. The important points are that success in one practice area contributes to success in another area, and that all the practices are informed by an attitude of mindfulness, as evidenced by:

- A more nuanced appreciation of context and ways to deal with it.
- Ongoing scrutiny of existing expectations.
- Continuous refinement and differentiation of expectations based on newer experiences.

- Willingness and capability to invent new expectations that make sense of unprecedented events.

- Identification of new dimensions of context that improve foresight and current functioning.

Table 2-1. The Mindful Organization: How the Attributes of Mindfulness Relate to the Four HRO Practices*	
Guiding HRO Practice	**Characteristic of a Mindful Organization (Sustaining HRO)**
1: Manage the System, Not the Parts • Ensure safety system selected provides safety • Manage the safety system to reduce variability • Foster a culture of reliability • Model organizational learning	*HROs anticipate the unexpected by being reluctant to simplify.* They: • Take deliberate steps to create more complete and nuanced pictures. • Simplify less and see more. This counteracts tendencies to simplify assumptions, expectations and analyses through practices such as adversarial reviews, selection of employees with nontypical prior experience, frequent job rotation, and retraining. • Know the world is complex, unstable, unknowable, and unpredictable, and position themselves to see as much as possible. They work to create a climate that encourages variety in people's analysis about the organization's technology and production processes, and establish practices that allow those perspectives to be heard and to make information visible that is not held in common.

Chapter 2 | 49

Table 2-1. The Mindful Organization: How the Attributes of Mindfulness Relate to the Four HRO Practices*

Guiding HRO Practice	Characteristic of a Mindful Organization (Sustaining HRO)
2: Reduce System Variability • Deploy the Break-the-Chain Safety Framework • Evaluate the operation of the safety system • Systematically adjust processes	*HROs anticipate the unexpected by being preoccupied with failure, that is, by having chronic unease.* They: • Encourage the reporting of errors. They work to create a climate where people feel safe to question assumptions and to report problems or failures candidly. They persuade their people to be chronically worried about the unexpected and sensitive to the fact that any decisions may be subject to faulty assumptions. • Elaborate experiences of near misses for what can be learned. Conduct reviews quickly before people have a chance to revise their stories and encourage close calls to be seen as failures that reveal potential danger rather than evidence of success. • Are wary of the potential liabilities of success, including complacency; the temptation to reduce margins of safety, and the drift into automatic processing. They create a climate where people are wary of success; suspicious of quiet periods; and concerned about stability, the routine, and the lack of challenge and variety that can lull an organization to relax its vigilance.

continued

50 | High Reliability Operations • A Practical Guide to Avoid the System Accident

Table 2-1. The Mindful Organization: How the Attributes of Mindfulness Relate to the Four HRO Practices*

Guiding HRO Practice	Characteristic of a Mindful Organization (Sustaining HRO)
3: Foster a Culture of Reliability • Enable employees to make conservative decisions • Ensure proficiency through hands-on-work • Encourage open questioning of and challenges to the safety system	*HROs contain the unexpected by deference to expertise.* They: • Cultivate diversity to notice more in complex environments (avoid rigid hierarchies). This encourages people to make knowledge about the system transparent and widely-known (the more people who know about system weaknesses and how to manage them, the faster they can notice and correct problems in the making). • Push decision-making to the front line, and allow authority to migrate to those with the most expertise, regardless of rank. This creates a set of operating dynamics that shifts leadership to the person who currently has the answer to the problem at hand (puts a premium on expertise over rank and allows decisions to migrate both downward and upward as conditions warrant). *HROs contain the unexpected by being committed to resilience.* They: • Demand deep knowledge of technology, systems, co-workers, self, and raw materials. They adopt an organization-wide mindset of cure rather than prevention in which the focus is on treating an anomaly, even before full diagnosis, to gain experience and a clearer picture of what they are treating. • Put a premium on experts with deep experience and skills and establish pockets of resilience by having uncommitted resources to solve sticky problems.

Chapter 2 | **51**

Table 2-1. The Mindful Organization: How the Attributes of Mindfulness Relate to the Four HRO Practices*

Guiding HRO Practice	Characteristic of a Mindful Organization (Sustaining HRO)
4: Learn and Adapt as an Organization • Generate decision-making information • Refine the HRO system: apply a system approach to reduce variability	*HROs anticipate the unexpected by being sensitive to operations.* They: • Don't wait for accidents to investigate latent organizational weaknesses; they know normal operations may provide "free lessons" that signal the development of unexpected events. As a result, they conduct incident reviews of unexpected results, no matter how inconsequential, and conduct reviews quickly before people revise their stories. • Employ situational awareness that allows continuous adjustments to prevent errors from accumulating and enlarging—they pay serious attention to operations, the front line, and imperfections in these features. • Notice anomalies while these are still tractable and can be isolated. • Know they cannot develop a big picture of operations if the symptoms are withheld. • Are concerned with the disconnect between operations as viewed from the top and as implemented on the front line. • Use operating practices that help people develop a collective cognitive map of operations at any one moment, such as situational assessments with continual updates and collective story-building about actual operations and workplace characteristics. *HROs contain the unexpected by being committed to resilience.* They: • Develop the capabilities to detect, contain, and bounce back from inevitable errors. • Pay as much attention to building capabilities to cope with errors as to improving capabilities to plan and anticipate events. • Work to keep errors small and improvise to keep the system functioning. • Develop capabilities for mindfulness, swift learning, flexible role structures, substitution and backup, and quick size-up.

*Weick and Sutcliffe, 2001

Chapter 3

Chapter 3

Transforming to an HRO: How to Develop a Guiding Strategy

This chapter answers the following questions:

- How does my organization develop a strategy for becoming an HRO?

- What are the seven elements used to drive a systems approach to transformation?

- How are the four HRO practices used to inform strategy development?

- How does my organization develop objectives and indicators?

- How does my organization measure the effectiveness of the transformation process?

Chapter 1 introduced the four guiding practices that characterize high reliability operations; Chapter 2 explained how you can use HRO Practice 1 as a tool to assimilate the other HRO practices into your operation. In essence, Chapter 2 provided a vision of the HRO end state; understanding and holding to this vision is the first step in the long process of transformation to an HRO. The second step is to develop a transformation strategy that will enable your operation to transition to an HRO. To help you in this endeavor, this chapter provides a hands-on process that will help you understand, plan, implement, and succeed in your organization's transformation.

The journey to become an HRO requires the same sort of strategic planning as any other organizational transformation. First, the strategic objectives are determined, and then a gap analysis is performed to determine the difference between the current state and the desired future state. Once the gaps are identified and measured, modified strategies with specific objectives, measures, targets, and initiatives are formulated. Figure 3-1 illustrates the six major steps of the transformation process.

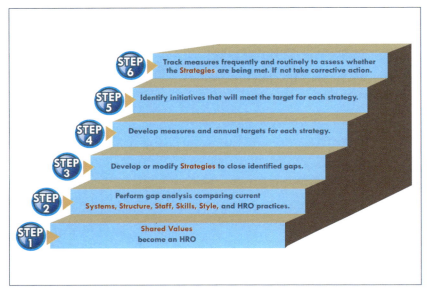

Figure 3-1. HRO Transformation Process

A Systems Approach to Strategic Planning

System events or accidents reveal weaknesses in the overall system of an organization. These weaknesses may be manifested in the structure of the organization itself, an incompatible business strategy, the wrong type of staff for the job at hand, a management style that does not stress high reliability, improper procedures or the failure of employees to follow procedures, a lack of communication, or a dozen other symptoms. The

McKinsey 7S approach, first published by Thomas J. Peters and Robert H. Waterman, Jr. in the book *In Search of Excellence* (1982), is a systematic tool for helping to expose and evaluate systemic weaknesses, imbalances, or incongruities. We apply the 7S approach to each HRO practice through the steps shown in Figure 3-1; this systematic approach ensures that every facet of business will be explicitly considered. As shown in Figure 3-2 (on the following page), the 7S approach uses seven interdependent variables to drive the analysis processes:

- Guiding concepts and *shared values* (i.e. culture)
- *Strategy*
- *Systems* and procedures
- *Structure*
- *Staff*
- Corporate strength and *skills*
- Management *style*

The beauty of this scheme is that it encourages managers embarking on change to realize that such change involves at least seven elements of complexity. This approach is particularly pertinent to organizations attempting to transform to HROs because—like the four practices we introduced in Chapter 1—it is based on a system approach that is mindful of the interdependencies of and need for balance among the various organizational attributes.

How does your organization begin the transformation to an HRO? Using Figure 3-1 as a guide, your first step is to ensure that *shared values* are in place. For the HRO journey, this shared value or vision is to *become an HRO* (as defined in Chapter 1 and further characterized in Chapter 2). The

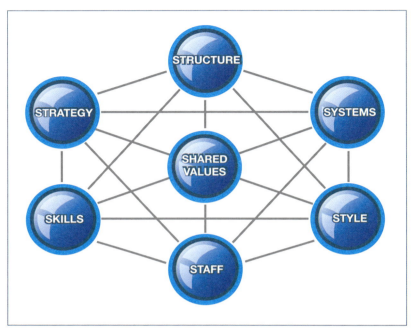

Figure 3-2. McKinsey 7S Approach for HRO Transformation (Peter and Waterman, 1982, p. 10)

specific strategies to be used to reach this overriding goal are determined in Step 2, the gap analysis. During this critical step, you must compare existing strategies, structure, systems, skills, style, and staff against the desired end state defined in Step 1. The identified gaps you identify between the current state of your organization and its desired end state help focus your attention on strategies to close these gaps (Step 3). Steps 4 and 5 help you develop performance measures, targets, and initiatives for each of these strategies.

The final step in the transformation process, Step 6, requires you to track and report against the developed measures to determine whether the strategies are succeeding. This is an important point: the measures selected are used to determine if a strategy is working, not that an initiative is finished. The initiatives should be designed to meet the performance target for a given strategy. In other words, you should use them to measure the effectiveness of the transformation process, not to indicate that the organization is functioning at the level of an HRO.

The six-step transformation is the same for every organization embarking on the HRO journey, but the individual prescriptions will vary depending on what the gap analysis reveals. Figure 3-3 shows that you should apply the 7S elements to each HRO practice to determine the gaps between current and ideal practices. This will allow you to develop strategies for each important element of complexity for each of the four HRO practices. For example, during their gap analysis of HRO Practice 1, Organization Alpha may find that its management structure and style is close to the desired practice, but that large gaps exist in other areas: management and technical skills, operating and feedback systems, and the alignment of certain staff assignments. Organization Beta may discover it lacks the proper organizational structure to support an HRO and needs to embark on a total overhaul of its operation. In either case, the organization would focus on their specific problem areas and develop strategies that will bring their operations more into alignment with the four HRO practices.

The next section of this chapter explains the 7S elements in more detail, followed by a discussion that explains how these elements can be used in combination with the four HRO practices to drive the transformation process. An example that illustrates how these strategies are applied and the metrics used to evaluate their success is included as the last section of the chapter.

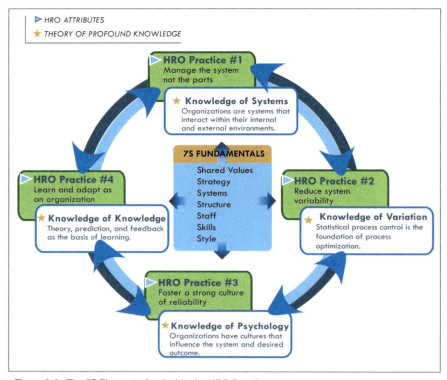

Figure 3-3. The 7S Elements Applied to the HRO Practices

The McKinsey 7S Approach: Seven Elements to Guide Your HRO Journey

The 7S approach focuses explicitly on both the hardware (strategy and structure) and the software (staff, style, systems, shared values, and skills) of an organization. It is critical that you consider each of the 7S elements during the gap analysis; whether or not your transformative strategies will embrace all seven elements or just a subset depends on the results of this analysis. Your organization must adapt the tactics and tools that will enable you to meet your transformational needs.

Shared Value

The shared value is the overriding goal of the organization—in this case, the desire to become an HRO as defined by the four HRO practices. HROs share a value (or vision) of excellence. They have earned the trust and confidence of the public as suppliers of goods or services that are dependable and safe. They have a clear vision of what success (safety and quality) looks like and strive to reach it every day through the use of concrete objectives and behaviors. Their measures, targets, and initiatives are clearly defined and align with their strategic goal and objectives. They have the gumption to stay the path. The leadership and employees are committed, not only to reach the end state, but to achieve their best every day of the journey. These shared values should permeate each of the HRO practices and inform the transformation process.

Strategy

Strategy is the organization's overall plan of action that will propel it from its current state to the desired end state. As defined in Chapter 1, an HRO is an organization that conducts relatively error-free operations over a long period of time. Inherent in this definition are the requirements of reliability and safety. Thus, HROs must provide excellent, dependable goods or services and—at the same time—make sure its employees, the environment, and the public are protected against a system accident. To prevent a system accident, an HRO must protect its high-hazard operations from the threat of human error. In other words, **greatly reducing or eliminating the opportunity for human error to trigger a series of events that may cascade into a system accident is an overriding strategy of an HRO.**

Based on the results of your gap analysis, you may have to modify existing strategies or develop additional strategies to close the gap between the existing and desired end state. These strategies will become the basis for the measures, targets, and initiatives that steer your organization along the path to becoming an HRO. Many consultants and texts are available for developing strategies and strategic plans, so it should not be too difficult to select a method that is appropriate for your organization. In the end, the method used is less important than ensuring that the strategies are well developed, clearly communicated, and well executed.

A good strategic plan is used for daily decision making and resource allocation. The strategies to transition to an HRO should be tethered by aggressive, but achievable goals. This combination of tactics and objectives becomes the basis on which priorities are set and decisions made. A good plan allows the organization to focus resources on strategic initiatives, and allows managers to justify their decisions to not fund initiatives, if they are not aligned with or supportive of the overall strategy. As a manager, you must guard against being seduced by good ideas that will divert funding and other resources from the defined strategy.

The Strategy-Focused Organization: How Balanced Scorecard Companies Thrive in the New Business Environment (2001), written by Robert Kaplan and David Norton, presents a process for flowing initiatives from an organization's overall vision and strategy. This process allows managers to focus on measuring the progress made toward achieving the strategy, rather than becoming distracted by checking off the completion of initiatives that, although useful, do not further the overall strategy. Kaplan and Norton (2001) indicate that most organizations use a backward approach to developing initiatives that looks something like this:

STRATEGY ▷ **INITIATIVES** ▷ **MEASURES**

This approach focuses the measures on whether or not an initiative was met, not whether the strategy is succeeding. Keep in mind that an initiative can be completed even though it does not help achieve, or even support, the strategy. For example, the human resources manager of your organization may determine it is time to upgrade the organization's major software system and initiates the steps to do so. The upgrade is completed and the efficiencies and timeliness of the upgrade is publicized throughout your organization. These are good business results; however, if the gap analysis did not indicate that upgrading this particular software system was of strategic importance to becoming an HRO, resources may have been diverted from other strategic initiatives for HRO transformation. Although this initiative was not inherently bad, it should not have been supported until the transformation to an HRO was complete and it was felt to be a necessary improvement towards operations at that point.

To avoid spending resources on initiatives that are not supportive of the overall strategy, Kaplan and Norton propose that managers should focus on an implementation process that looks like this:

STRATEGY ▷ **OBJECTIVE** ▷ **MEASURES** ▷ **TARGET** ▷ **INITIATIVES**

This process ties initiatives directly to strategy through a systematic approach that (1) determines how the objectives that support the strategy will be measured, (2) sets goals or targets for moving toward the objective, and (3) develops and implements initiatives that will support the first year's target.

Implementing strategy is a journey, not a destination. The strategy to become an HRO should transcend years of tactical operations and long-range plans that merely extend the current operating philosophy. Becoming an HRO is about fundamental change—transforming into a different sort of organization altogether. This may take several years, depending on where your organization is currently located along a continuum that extends from normal operations—as embodied in the concept of Perrow's Normal Accident Theory (1999)—to high reliability operations. Each year, you should update initiatives to reflect progress (or lack of it), but the basic strategy should not change. Objectives should be modified only after they have been met and the organization has moved from the planning and transformational stage of the journey to the implementing and sustaining stage.

System

As discussed in Chapter 1, a systems approach is needed to avoid the consequential accident. A system may include many things—operating procedures, communication, inventory, transportation, engineering, process design, maintenance, document control, safety, and quality are only some of the components that can make up a system. A transformation strategy must ensure that all systems and components are supportive of the vision and do not have independent and competing objectives.

Chapter 3 | **63**

Management behavior, such as underfunding or understaffing an operation, is frequently a contributing cause to system events or accidents. A key focus, therefore, is to ensure that all supporting systems are well-designed and in balance with one another. For example, an inventory system that relies on just-in-time delivery is incompatible with a procurement system that requires a lengthy ordering and approval process. Likewise, a document management system that requires many approvals and a long queue time is unsuited for use with an operating process that requires the ability to revise procedures rapidly to avoid production downtime.

Systems are arguably the most important aspect of an HRO. The systems used by an HRO must be designed, deployed, and used in a manner that support high reliability operations and provides feedback to determine if there has been practical drift, or the unintentional movement of the organization away from system controls over time.

Measurement and feedback data can come from a variety of sources and can take many forms to include management assessments, internal audits, root cause analysis investigations of events, process improvement initiatives, and business health indicators. Your goal is to select metrics that will predict and prevent accidents through the use of realistic performance indicators, trend analysis, and rapid correction of issues. Accumulate useful data in a form that can be used, analyzed, and acted upon.

Finally, an HRO needs an effective corrective action program to correct system problems. You must monitor corrective actions derived from findings and incidents, and even from improvement initiatives, to determine the following:

- Is the action appropriate for the finding?

- Does the action resolve systemic issues or is it a quick fix?

- Does the problem indicate a negative trend? That is, is this a repeat occurrence or a variation on previous incidents or findings? If so, the systemic solution may not yet have been found and implemented.

- Are actions completed and closed out (as opposed to merely closed out)?

- Do all parties responsible for corrective actions know about the proposed actions and agree to the scope, deliverables, and cost?

- Is the corrective action plan funded?

Structure

A poor organizational structure can be just as detrimental to a system as technical or operational failures, yet little has been published about the relationship between organizational structure and high reliability operations. Because an organization is a system, the organizational structure can greatly influence the effectiveness of all other initiatives. The structure must be consistent with the management style and HRO operating systems; a structure that does not support these elements may, unobtrusively but persistently, stymie any efforts to meet strategic objectives. For instance, an organization that designs its processes on a staff matrix basis, but funds resources on a hierarchical basis, may unwittingly and negatively affect the success of projects that draw resources from support organizations. Likewise, initiatives or objectives that require fast response and decision making may languish or be derailed in organizations with tightly controlled, hierarchical authority. It makes no sense to send a

Chapter 3 **65**

staff representative to a meeting about an urgent matter if only the senior leadership is empowered to make decisions.

Organizational structure can exert a powerful, though inconspicuous, influence on the success or failure of strategies. Structure alone is not the key to a strategy's success, but if your organization's structure is not aligned with the HRO practices, it can cause the HRO transformation to fail.

Staff

Staff refers to the characteristics of members of the organization as well as to their allocation and deployment. An HRO must be properly staffed. Clearly, line operations must have adequate staff to perform the business functions. In addition, adequate numbers of qualified and certified safety professionals should be available to ensure safety in all applicable areas, whether the danger is from chemicals, explosives, radiation, industrial processes, industrial hygiene, occupational medicine, biohazards, or other factors. Make sure that safety resources are allocated to the line operations they support, that they work as part of the team, and that they support your organizational strategy to become an HRO.

Make sure that your support staff are adequately trained and allocated as needed. Support personnel are part of the overall team; an HRO must recognize this by providing adequate supplies, material, tools, and personnel, and by recognizing the accomplishments of support staff as well as line operators when accolades are given for meeting production goals. Support staff includes engineers, scientists, work planners, material handlers, and—of special importance—plant maintenance personnel. Your organization cannot expect to become an HRO if the facility (or facilities) has excessive deferred maintenance or the equipment is not operating at peak efficiency. Such conditions foster a culture that relies on a "make do" approach, which can lead to practical drift and, eventually, to a system accident.

Staff members at every level of your organization should be able to attain a high level of job satisfaction. All employees should feel challenged and remain sufficiently busy, but should not be so stretched by competing demands that they are tempted to cut corners. Ideally, each employee should feel they accomplished something important and worthwhile every day.

Skills

Skills are those distinctive abilities that set people and their organizations apart from the competition. HRO employees must have the technical skills to design, operate, understand, and continuously improve the operation of their organization. This requires excellence in science and technology coupled with sound operational design. All employees must understand the unique hazards associated with their operation and respect those hazards. To achieve and maintain this high level of operation and awareness, training and education must be a paramount and continuous characteristic of an HRO. Training to ensure basic job skills as well as to cultivate proficiency in problem solving, investigative tools such as Causal Factors Analysis, and tools used to analyze feedback data should supplement continuous technical training. Make sure that training is focused, of high quality, and appropriate to meet strategic objectives. Resources should not be expended on training that does not add value or support the organizational objectives.

Style

Style is a description of how managers such as yourself execute their functions as emphasized in HRO Practice 1—their commitment, perseverance, enthusiasm, courage, and decisiveness (or their lack of these traits). The commitment to become an HRO cannot be treated lightly by managers. Lip service is not adequate; this not an initiative that can be announced and then brushed under the carpet so that business can go on as usual. It must be a campaign that is attended to each and every day by all managers and employees. Only an inspired top leader can make that happen.

The enthusiasm of the organization's top leader for becoming an HRO and sustaining high reliability operations must go beyond commitment—it must teeter on the brink of zealotry. The leader must not waiver from his path and must be courageous enough to establish both a culture of reliability and all the supporting systems. This requires commitment of resources, consistent decision making that supports the shared values and vision to become an HRO, and the backbone to replace or reassign managers who fail to share that vision. A leader must be willing to stay with the organization long enough to see it through this transformation.

In addition to an inspired top leader, an HRO needs managers whose management style encourages accountability and openness; employees must not fear to report problems or difficulties because of a real or perceived danger of retribution. The organizational culture must value honesty and the exposure of systemic problems by supporting, not punishing, employees who provide feedback. This is critical for fostering an atmosphere in which employees and the organization as a whole can learn from mistakes and implement corrective actions. At the same time, each employee must take ownership and responsibility to ensure safe operations, and line managers must set examples as servant leaders, that is, they should make the needs and priorities of their employees a top priority (Greenleaf, 1977). There should be mutual respect between management and employees at every level. Communication should flow freely in all directions, and managers should foster an excellent spirit of teamwork.

Using the Four HRO Practices to Inform Strategy Development

As shown in Figure 3-1, the 7S elements should be applied throughout the six-step process, particularly during Steps 1 and 2. The key is to use the 7S elements as heuristics to compare an organization's current operations to the four HRO practices. In essence, your goal is to take a snapshot of where your organization currently lies on the continuum between normal—as indicated in Perrow's Normal Accident Theory (1999)—and HRO operations for each of the HRO practices (Figure 3-3). The 7S elements provide the backdrop that brings the snapshot into focus.

This concept is best illustrated with an actual example. The following section describes the process used by a hypothetical high-hazard operation in its effort to become an HRO. Notice how the organization uses the 7S elements to guide the process, and then focuses on the problem areas to devise transformative strategies.

How to Apply the 7S Approach: An Illustrative Example

Company Alpha is in a high-hazard industry that has managed and operated the same plant for over 50 years. It experienced one catastrophic accident, 30 years ago, that resulted in a fatality and the loss of a facility. As a result of that accident, operation facilities were brought up to new safety standards, and training and procedures were upgraded to improve the safety of all operations. In addition, Company Alpha embraced the philosophy of the U.S. Department of Energy's Conduct of Operations (U.S. DOE, Order 5480.19) 15 years ago, and embarked on a concerted effort to increase operational safety to a much more reliable state. This included a significant investment in procedure improvement, tooling redesign and deployment, training for all of the workforce, and even replacement of key management positions to institute the new culture. Overall, Company Alpha is well-respected in the industry, well-run, and has operated with only a few minor safety or procedural incidents since the Conduct of Operations was institutionalized. In fact, Company Alpha is considered world class for employee safety, receiving an award last year for being one of the safest workplaces in the country. Nevertheless, because Company Alpha is in a high-hazard business, it is very concerned for the safety of its employees, the community, and the environment; therefore, Company Alpha desires to transform into an HRO.

To begin the transformation, the general manager sponsored a series of seminars for key senior and mid-level managers to learn about the practices and attributes of HROs. These seminars were also used to pilot a new CFA process that emphasizes methods for identifying and learning from information-rich, low-consequence events as a means of ferreting out and correcting problem areas that could lead to the Big One. The general manager felt passionate enough about the topic

---

Conduct Of Operations

The philosophy associated with any operation must include the deliberate application of controls and methods to ensure safe, compliant, and productive operation of the facility or activity. Conduct of Operations, sometimes referred to as "formality of operations," is the application of that philosophy.

(U.S. DOE, Order 5480.19)

to teach several seminars himself, and encouraged each of the senior staff members to teach at least a portion of the seminars. Each seminar attendee was provided books to read on HROs and culture, and also reviewed past incident reports and events for lessons learned. Concurrent with the training, the new CFA process was applied to several information-rich, low-consequence system events so that the various tools could be tested on actual investigations and the overall process optimized.

With the groundwork laid, the next step in the transformation is to develop strategies to institute HRO practices that may still need improvement. Company Alpha is following the six-step process presented earlier in this chapter to transform into an HRO; the process is informed by the 7S approach in combination with the HRO practices.

Step 1: Establish Shared Values
This step has already been taken by Company Alpha. The desire to become an HRO is strong; the effort is spearheaded by the general manager, who has ensured that training has been provided to key senior and mid-level managers. A CFA process has emerged that suits the needs of the organization.

Step 2: Perform Gap Analysis
This is the most difficult step. It involves comparing the current structure, systems, skills, style, and staff of the organization to those identified as essential to support the four HRO practices. This step is broken down into its components in the following discussion.

Structure. Company Alpha has a traditional hierarchical organizational structure that is separated into functional units called divisions. Each division is led by a division manager who reports to the general manager, and is divided into smaller departments. Departments are further subdivided into sections, depending on their size or function. The number of departments and sections in each division are determined at the discretion of the division manager, which indicates some level of flexibility in organizational design; however, the flexibility is fairly limited. Company Alpha has been organized this way since its inception, so this structure is well ingrained into the culture of the organization, and also is reflected in many operating policies and procedures including funding allocation, document management, and communication protocols. Although projects are considered to operate cross functionally, there is still a noticeable preference by project team members to respond to priorities set by their functional manager in lieu of delivering in accordance with a project schedule.

After comparing the current organizational structure to the attributes of an HRO, Company Alpha concluded that its overall structure generally suits its operation. The production work is the outcome of divisions aligned to either perform or provide support for production. Company Alpha realizes that important initiatives— including preparation for operational readiness reviews—are managed through projects, and the company is committed to good project management. The management team agrees that project support should be elevated. Thus, one strategy that Company Alpha will pursue in their transformation process will be to provide increased support and priority for project deliverables.

Systems. Because of the high risk nature of the work Company Alpha performs, there are many rigorous systems in place to control the work. These include production planning, scheduling, and performance; procedure development, review, and publication; configuration management of tooling, structures, systems, and components; performance assurance and internal audits; management development including in-house training and educational assistance; maintenance work control; occurrence reporting and CFA; long-range and strategic planning; supply chain management; transportation and material handling; program and project management; safety of the employee, plant, and environment including waste management; budget planning and execution; and human resource management. These systems are mature and have undergone numerous internal and external assessments and audits over the years. Taking an honest look at the systems, Company Alpha concludes the following:

- Work control practices are very robust and drive consistent and desired results. The frequency of procedural noncompliance is remarkably low. In addition, the cycle time for production and maintenance is short.

- Company Alpha underwent an initiative several years ago to substitute nonhazardous material in work processes and has held close control against negative creep in this area.

- Engineered safety controls are the standard in process design and are extended to the design of production tooling, electronic testers, and every production procedure. Administrative controls are few and an ongoing program to evaluate the safety basis for operation continues to work to eliminate these.

- Company Alpha has a strong quality program. Its product is required to meet extremely tight standards or the customer will not accept it. In fact, the customer maintains offices at the production facility, where, in addition to performing quality acceptance activities, it is an integral part of the quality assurance process.

- Human error has been designed out of the process to a great extent. A complicated and comprehensive set of checks and balances, including multiple person review and engineered redundancy, provides Company Alpha confidence that mitigation against human error is well-controlled. The company realizes it is impossible to eradicate human error entirely; nevertheless, many layers of barriers are in place.

- Rigorous performance standards are established and enforced in safety, regulatory compliance, and nuclear safety.

- Facilities are a concern. The plant has been in continuous operation for over 50 years. It underwent one episode of significant new construction after the catastrophic accident and is currently undergoing a campaign to reduce the deferred maintenance backlog. Company Alpha believes this is an area of vulnerability and determines that a strategy for the funding and management of facility maintenance is needed to eliminate the growth of deferred maintenance altogether.

- Although there is a wealth of data on production performance, lessons learned, performance assurance assessments and audits, continuous improvement initiatives, and safety performance, this information is held in separate databases. The databases are not integrated, not easily accessible, and not routinely reviewed to look for trends, precursors, or indicators of any kind. Company Alpha recognizes it needs to use this data to look for indication of negative or troubling performance trends. In addition, the company needs a user-friendly method of turning the data into information, which can then be transformed into knowledge. A strategic initiative to improve knowledge captured from collected data is required, along with a strategy to take action and provide feedback on both negative and positive data trends.

Skills. Company Alpha has many job categories that are designated as requiring critical skills and has an extensive training program for production employees as well as for management. A relatively new software system to track the training and qualification levels of many jobs has been judged adequate by a recent external assessment. After a comprehensive review of skills required for high reliability operations, Company Alpha concludes that training in problem solving and systems thinking is needed for all employees. A strategy to develop and deploy these skills to all employees is required.

Management Style. Company Alpha's general manager is committed to transforming the company into an HRO and has taken decisive steps to lead the organization in that direction. An initial series of seminars has been delivered to selected senior and mid-level managers and the CFA process has been fine tuned and deployed in several incident investigations. Even so, an overall vision has not been fully imparted to the entire work force and there has been no training for the managers who did not attend the first series of seminars. An education and training campaign for all employees is required to instill the shared value of becoming an HRO; this campaign should also encourage more frequent use of the CFA process for analyzing information-rich, low-consequence events.

Company Alpha has a very strong culture that will be an advantage on its journey to become an HRO. The attrition rate among production and production support employees is very low and the employees enjoy an excellent salary and benefit package. Many employees have family members who also work for Company Alpha, some of them as far back as three generations. This leads to a real sense of community among the workforce and engenders a feeling of shared pride in their work. Because of the hazardous nature of the work, the plant is more than 20 miles from the nearest city, and more than 10 miles from the closest community of any size. This results in numerous car pools and lunch groups that strengthen friendships and often last for decades. The employees are mindful of the hazards of the work they perform and safety is valued by the entire workforce. As a result, Company Alpha's management is quite confident there will be support for this new vision. They believe the management style of an HRO is already in place.

Staff. Company Alpha has an experienced management staff, many of whom have spent most of their careers working in high-hazard industries or the military. All divisions are adequately staffed with the exception of the maintenance division, which is under its approved staffing level by 50 crafts persons. A strategic initiative to hire to the approved staffing level in the appropriate skill mix is required.

Although the other divisions are adequately staffed, Company Alpha recognizes it has difficulty retaining engineers, scientists, and information technology (IT) professionals. The staffing level is adequate, but the experience base is suffering because many of these employees leave Company Alpha with less than five years of service. A strategy to improve job retention for engineers, scientists, and IT professionals is required.

Step 3: Develop or Modify Strategies to Close Identified Gaps

In addition to the strategies identified through the gap analysis, Company Alpha already had long-term strategies in place for improving operational excellence in three areas:

- Superior teamwork

- Superior work planning, execution, and control

- Superior sustained and reliable production

These strategies are already being deployed and, because they are supportive of the vision to become an HRO, they will continue. The strategies that were derived from the gap analysis are as follows:

- Support the priority for project deliverables in addition to production deliverables.

- Stop the growth of deferred maintenance.

- Institute knowledge capture methods to facilitate organizational learning.

- Institute a method to distill knowledge in actionable continuous improvement initiatives, including feedback of negative and positive trends to management and operations.

- Increase maintenance division staffing to the approved staffing level and in the appropriate skill mix.

Chapter 3

- Develop and deploy problem-solving and systems thinking skills to all employees.

- Deploy an education and training campaign for all employees on the vision to become an HRO.

- Institutionalize the use of the CFA process for information-rich, low-consequence events.

- Improve job retention for engineers, scientists, and IT professionals.

Company Alpha sets a goal to be fully transformed into an HRO in five years. This allows a phased approach that may be supported by the financial plan, and also allows gradual but steady institutionalization of new programs.

Step 4: Develop Measures and Annual Targets for Each Strategy and

Step 5: Identify Initiatives That Will Meet the Target for Each Strategy

For each strategy identified in Steps 2 and 3, Company Alpha needs to establish a measure, a target or targets for that measure, and initiatives to reach those targets. The difficulty here is that the measures must ensure that the strategy is being implemented successfully, not indicate that an initiative is completed. Likewise, the initiatives must focus on meeting annual targets. When all initiatives are completed and the targets for each measure have been met, the strategy will be fully in place. It is possible for there to be more than one measure for a strategy, and the targets may change over the five-year implementation period.

The senior management team is assigned this task, with the general manager retaining oversight and final approval. The general manager is committed to ensuring the strategies are completed in five years, so the strategies need to be aggressive but attainable. Some strategies will be completed in less than five years. Examples of measures, targets, and initiatives for Company Alpha's first three implementing strategies are provided in Table 3-1.

Step 6: Track Measures Frequently and Routinely to Assess Whether Strategies Are Being Met

With strategies, measures, targets, and initiatives established, Company Alpha now needs to assign senior manager sponsors for each strategy, and ensure the initiatives are funded and staffing is assigned to execute them. Status needs to be provided to the general manager on a routine basis, and corrections to targets or initiatives made as the process continues and feedback is received.

Company Alpha is now ready to proceed with the transformation to an HRO. Despite the company's high level of safety consciousness and strong culture, the transformation is a daunting task that will require commitment of resources and time to accomplish in the five-year window established by the general manager. Care must be taken to ensure that the company does not lose its strategic focus as time passes; execution of these strategies must remain a priority despite other pressures. The strength and commitment of the general manager and senior team will be tested, but Company Alpha has successfully effected other major transformations in the past and is confident it will ultimately achieve its vision to become an HRO.

Chapter 3 | 79

Table 3-1. Company Alpha Strategies, Measures, and Targets

Strategy	Measure	Target	Initiatives
Support the priority for project deliverables in addition to production deliverables.	Decrease project schedule delays due to missed functional support deliverables.	Year 1: establish baseline based on past 3 years projects Year 2: reduce from baseline by 50% Year 3: reduce from baseline by 75% Year 4: reduce from baseline by 100%	Add project deliverables and milestones to the weekly production planning meeting agenda. Include project manager input in annual performance reviews.
Stop the growth of deferred maintenance.	Dollar value of deferred maintenance backlog FCI = DM/Plant Replacement Value (goal is <5%).	Year 1: establish DM backlog and FCI baseline Year 2: reduce DM backlog by 30% from baseline Year 3: reduce DM backlog by 30% from baseline Year 4: reduce DM backlog by 30% from baseline Year 5: FCI <5%	Year 1: Perform plant-wide condition assessment survey (CAS) data to establish deferred maintenance (DM) backlog. Package DM into upgrade projects. Years 2 – 4: Execute upgrade projects. Justify increased funding for base maintenance such that DM backlog is not developed. Institute CAS inspection program such that entire plant is reviewed every three years. Year 5: Develop funding plan to sustain plant at current facility condition index (FCI).

continued

Table 3-1. Company Alpha Strategies, Measures, and Targets

Strategy	Measure	Target	Initiatives
Institute knowledge capture methods to facilitate organizational learning.	Repeat occurrences with same systemic cause.	Year 1: establish baseline trend data for causal factors Year 2: reduce from baseline by 50% Year 3: reduce from baseline by 75% Year 4: reduce from baseline by 100%	Years 1 and 2: review data from all sources (audits, assessments, CFA, Six Sigma projects, etc.) and perform analysis to determine repeat problems. Perform causal loop analysis to determine systemic solutions for most significant causes. Assign information manager to develop a system to take data and distill information. Develop decision support system that co-locates results of information for management knowledge capture. Years 3 – 5: Develop and execute initiatives for systemic solutions determined from causal loop analysis.

CAS = condition assessment survey   DM = deferred maintenance   FCI = facility condition index

Chapter 4

Chapter 4

Break the Chain Between Threat and Hazard: A Safety System Framework

This chapter answers the following questions:

- What are the six common pitfalls that an HRO must avoid?

- What does it mean to break the chain from threat to hazard?

- How does the Break-the-Chain Framework relate to the four HRO practices?

- What are the six steps of the Break-the-Chain Framework?

- How can my organization evaluate its safety system and adjust its processes?

In Chapter 1, we stated that a system accident, which has devastating consequences, occurs when an operational hazard is threatened by (and vulnerable to) human error, and indicated that one of the major goals of an HRO is to prevent a system accident (and its associated consequences). We introduced the four major HRO practices in Chapter 1, and discussed HRO Practice 1, which depends on transparent and mindful management, in Chapter 2. In Chapter 3, we provided guidelines for organizational transformation using a systematic approach to develop strategies, initiatives, and performance indicators.

This chapter—and the remaining chapters in this guide—focus on tools and methodologies that will help your organization implement and

FAA Safety Culture

The Federal Aviation Agency came under heavy fire today as the chairman of the House Transportation And Infrastructure Committee accused the agency of "the most serious lapse in safety . . . in the past 23 years" and threatened to break up what he called "a culture of coziness" between senior agency officials and the airlines they are tasked with regulating. "The committee's investigation uncovered a pattern of regulatory abuse and widespread regulatory lapses that allowed 117 aircraft to be operated in commercial service despite being out of compliance with airworthiness directors," Chairman James Oberstar (D-Minn) said. "FAA needs to clean house, from the top down."

(Neuman, 2008)

sustain operations as an HRO. Each of the tools we present is dependent upon and informed by the four HRO practices and has been tested at our own organization. But there is nothing sacred about the systems and methods we present; we encourage you to adapt them to fit your own operations and the needs of your organization.

In this chapter, we first present six common pitfalls that can lead to system accidents. We then introduce an HRO safety system designed to address these pitfalls. We call this system the Break-the-Chain Framework because it is designed to sever the links that lead from the threat (human error) to the operational hazard.

We believe the Break-the-Chain Framework is effective (that is, it is properly designed to protect against physical operational hazards) if it is enforced and adhered to by all members of an organization. To avoid a high-consequence accident, however, you and other managers and employees must continually monitor and strive to minimize any variation from the system as designed—and to be on the lookout for design flaws. Thus, you will ensure operational safety and reliability through continued refinement of the safety system, organizational learning, and the development of a culture of reliability.

Common Pitfalls that Can Lead to System Accidents

As we have pointed out many times, sustaining HRO practices is every bit as difficult as the journey to become an HRO—if not more so. This section identifies common operational pitfalls that, if left unchecked, could result in a system accident. Figure 4-1 shows where these failures typically occur in the chain that leads from threat to hazard.

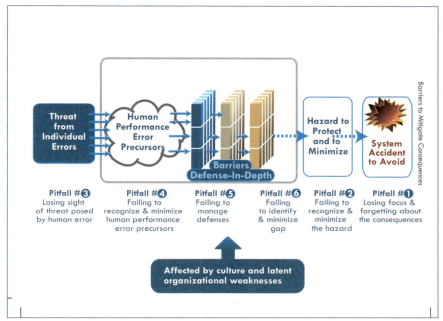

Figure 4-1. The Break-the-Chain Framework

These common pitfalls are identified for two reasons. First, they provide an organization with insight into what can go wrong. This knowledge is critical to system designers, organizational leaders, operational managers, and safety officers because it helps them look for and correct these deficiencies before they result in a system accident. In this respect, the pitfalls presented here illustrate the logic behind the Break-the-Chain Framework we describe later in this chapter, which is designed to prevent these pitfalls. Second, they provide insight into how to conduct an event investigation if an unplanned event does occur (read more about this in Chapter 6).

Pitfall 1. Losing Focus and Forgetting About the Consequences

As discussed in Chapter 1, a primary discriminator between system accidents and other types of accidents and events is the severity of the consequence and the number of victims. No organization wants to have a catastrophic accident. Yet, in the course of many accident investigations, it becomes clear that employees involved in the events leading to the accident often lost sight of why safety precautions were so critical to their operation. Edwin Zebroski, in a 2003 presentation on the attributes of seven major accidents, noted that **one of the most common attributes associated with major accidents is the mindset that success is routine.** He quotes one official as saying "No serious accidents [have occurred] in my 23 years with this organization. Why worry about unlikely things?" According to Zebroski, this attitude is typical among many organization officials when being investigated after accidents.

Luckily, catastrophic accidents do not occur often in high-hazard operations. This is good, but it also makes it more difficult for an HRO to keep its focus. It is normal for humans to feel safe and forget about the consequences of an accident when a long period of time has passed without a major event; the problem is that a feeling of safety will naturally lead to complacency, and complacent employees may lose the motivation to maintain and support safety systems. Resources may be diverted to other corporate objectives and the supporting safety infrastructure (human, physical, and mechanical) can degrade. Too frequently, complacency leads to what Diane Vaughan (CAIB, 2003) terms *normalized deviance*, which is the tendency to redefine and accept previously unexpected anomalies over time as

Chapter 4 | **85**

expected events and, ultimately, as acceptable risks (U.S. DOE, 2007).[6] This in turn, makes it much easier for a system accident to occur.

Pitfall 2: Failing to Recognize and Minimize the Hazard

What you don't know can hurt you. Failure to recognize hazards is the first step in the recipe for disaster. The second step is failure to maintain a chronic unease concerning these identified hazards (Figure 4-1). Even the most hazardous materials can become routine to employees who have never experienced a near-miss or consequential event. This can lead to a blasé attitude about handling hazardous materials and using standard operating procedures meant to ensure safety. Practical drift creeps into the operation.

High-hazard operations court disaster when they choose not to take steps—such as the substitution of less hazardous materials, the physical separation of hazardous materials from possible initiators or catalysts, or the reduction of hazardous materials stored in any one location—any of which would minimize operational hazards and the consequences associated with a system accident. Most organizations fail to reduce their physical hazards because of the costs involved. For example, the cost associated with substituting less hazardous chemicals for the ones currently in use may be perceived as too expensive. This is particularly common when an organization has a good safety record and perceives the risk to be less than the cost of mitigation. This demonstrates how complacency may prevent an organization from exploring new ways to reduce its operational hazards.

Organizations may also fail to minimize hazards because they do not recognize how changes to the design and management of their operations could decrease the likelihood of a system accident (or they recognize this, yet still fail to make the changes). In Chapter 1, we discussed how a nuclear reactor represents a system with complex and tightly-coupled interactions, and indicated that such interactions could make an operation more prone to system accidents. This example, which involves mechanical systems, illustrates how disaster can occur when conditions change so quickly that an operator cannot take appropriate actions to avert disaster (e.g., Chernobyl Nuclear Facility, 1986). The fact is, interactive complexity and tight coupling are relative terms that are dependent on the speed of the organization to recognize and respond to errors, negative trends, and inconsequential events (weak signals or symptoms). The slower the organization's ability to recognize and respond, the tighter the effective coupling of the system, and hence the greater the probability that small incidents will escalate to consequential events. Yet many organizations do not know how much time it would take for their operation to respond to a critical situation, which leaves them without the proper controls to avoid pending accidents.

Pitfall 3: Losing Sight of the Threat Posed by Human Error

As described in Chapter 1, human error is typically considered the major threat to an operational hazard, whether it be a nuclear reactor, chemical stockpile, or supersonic aircraft (Figure 4-1). Human or individual error is universal—no one is immune from error regardless of age, experience, or educational level. Consequently, errors will happen. No amount of counseling, training, or motivation can alter a person's fallibility. Dr. James Reason, author of *Human Error* (1990) states that,

"It is crucial that personnel and particularly their managers become more aware of the human potential for errors; the task, workplace, and organizational factors that shape their likelihood; and their consequences. Understanding how and why unsafe acts occur is the essential first step in effective error management" (U.S. DOE, 2007).

Failing to understand human error makes us victims to its effects. Human errors occur for various reasons. According to the DOE *Human Performance Handbook* (2007), human error can be broken down into three performance modes—skill-based, rule-based, or knowledge-based—each of which can lead to different types and rates of error. Figure 4-2 illustrates how these three performance modes reflect an employee's various degrees of familiarity with a task, and thus, the amount of attention that is given to the task. Brief descriptions of each of these performance modes and the associated errors are provided on the following pages.

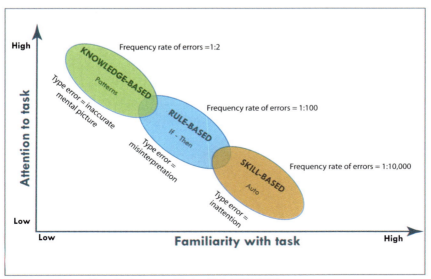

Figure 4-2. Human Error Performance Modes (U.S. DOE, 2007)

Skill-Based Mode

This performance mode involves highly practiced, often physical actions in familiar situations. Actions are usually executed from memory and behavior is governed by preprogrammed instructions developed through training or experience. Skills may become automatic over time, thus the major type of error in skill-based performance is inattention. Skill-based errors are primarily execution errors, typically triggered by human variability or by failure to recognize changes in task requirements, system response, or facility conditions related to the task. The expected error rate in skill-based mode is on the order of 1 in 10,000.

Rule-Based Mode

Employees move from a skill-based performance mode to a rule-based mode to deal with situational changes that require them to make conscious behavioral choices. They are likely dealing with a problem they have encountered before, have been trained to deal with, or which is covered by the procedures. Memorized or written rules are applied to the situation using an "if, then" logic, and conscious thinking may be used to verify whether this solution is appropriate. The prevalent type of error is misinterpretation. Errors involve deviating from an approved procedure, applying the wrong response to a work situation, or applying the correct procedure to the wrong situation. The expected error rate in rule-based mode is on the order of 1 in 100.

Knowledge-Based Mode

Employees enter the knowledge-based performance mode when they are uncertain about what to do. If uncertainty is high, the need for information becomes paramount (Turner and Pidgeon, 1997) and attention becomes more focused (Wickens, 1992). Knowledge-based situations are puzzling and involve patchy or inaccurate understanding (patterns) with conflicting, excessive, or inadequate data. Stress is usually high, as are the demands on the information-processing capabilities of the individual. Often, decisions are made with limited information and faulty assumptions. Consequently, the prevalent error type is an inaccurate mental image of the system, process, or facility status. The chance for error is particularly high, approximately 1 in 2 (50 percent) to 1 in 10 (Reason, 1997).

Pitfall 4: Failing to Recognize and Minimize Human Performance Error Precursors

The fourth potential pitfall common to high-hazard operations involves failing to identify and to reduce the *human performance error precursors* that increase *error-likely situations* (Figure 4-1). Human performance error precursors are unfavorable conditions embedded in the operation that create mismatches between a task and the individual. Error precursors interfere with successful performance and increase the probability for error. Simply stated, they are conditions that create error-likely situations, or error traps (Reason, 1997).

Human performance error precursors can be organized into one or more of the following four categories (U.S. DOE, 2007):

- *Task demands* are specific mental, physical, and team requirements needed to perform an activity that may either exceed the capabilities or challenge the limitations of the individual assigned to the task. Task demands include physical demands, task difficulty, and complexity. Examples include excessive workload, time pressures, concurrent actions, unclear roles and responsibilities, and vague standards.

- *Individual capabilities* are the unique mental, physical, and emotional characteristics of a particular person that fail to match the demands of the specific task. This involves cognitive and physical limitations such as unfamiliarity with the task, unsafe attitudes, level of education, lack of knowledge, unpracticed skills, personality, inexperience, health and fitness issues, poor communication practices, fatigue, and low self-esteem.

- *Work environment* includes general influences of the workplace such as organizational and cultural conditions that affect individual behavior. These include distractions, awkward equipment layout, complex tag out procedures, at-risk norms and values, work group attitudes toward various hazards, work control processes, and temperature, lighting, and noise.

- *Human nature* represents generic traits, dispositions, and limitations that may incline individuals to err under unfavorable conditions. Habit, short-term memory, stress, complacency, inaccurate risk perception, mind-set, and mental shortcuts are all examples of human nature.

A failure to recognize human performance error precursors results in both an increased number of errors and an increased vulnerability of the system.

Pitfall 5: Failing to Manage Defenses
The fifth pitfall is a failure to manage the defenses put in place to avoid the system accident (Figure

4-1). High-hazard operations typically design redundant barriers or *defenses-in-depth* into their systems to provide overlapping protection against a system accident. Yet there is no such thing as a complete defense. Every defense or barrier possesses holes and gaps created by *latent conditions* within the organization. All organizations possess latent conditions, which represent circumstances that result from management decisions that may have inadvertent and delayed effects on the integrity of various layers of defenses. For example, say your company commits to a very aggressive production schedule for the upcoming year. Unfortunately, the process efficiencies that you were expecting to come through did not materialize and you are unable to accomplish all your work if you follow the cumbersome operational process (your company's designed defense against hazards). The pressure on you to make your quota is mounting and you feel an urge to cut some corners. After all, you've skipped a few steps in the procedure before and nothing bad has happened. But wait! Your organization's operational defenses have just been undermined by a latent condition (pressure to make your quota) that manifested itself in an active error (failure to follow standard procedures). Such latent conditions create holes and gaps in organizational barriers, technical barriers or human barriers, thus opening a window of opportunity that allows the threat (individual error) to make damaging contact with the hazard (Figure 4-3 on the following page).

A system accident can also occur when one or more defenses fail. Such a failure typically indicates that the barrier did not serve its original purpose or that it was circumvented or penetrated by active failures (errors and violations committed by front-line personnel). Some common flaws

> **Latent Conditions**
>
> Hidden deficiencies in management control processes or values that create workplace conditions that can provoke errors (precursors) and degrade the integrity of defenses (flawed defenses).
>
> *(U.S. DOE, 2007)*

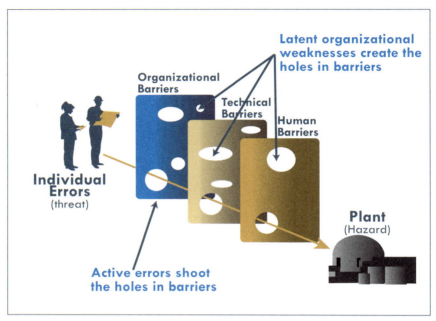

Figure 4-3. Defeating Defense-in-Depth: Effect of Active and Latent Errors on Barriers (Reason, 1997)

> **Active versus Latent Error**
>
> Active error is human action (behavior) that changes equipment, system, or plant state triggering immediate undesired consequences.
>
> Latent error is an error, act, or decision that results in organization-related weaknesses or equipment flaws that lie dormant until revealed either by human error, testing, or self-assessment.
>
> *(U.S. DOE, 2007)*

with engineered defenses that challenge employee performance and can contribute to system events and accidents include:

- Out-of-service equipment, controls, alarms, and indicators
- Workarounds, temporary repairs, or long-term temporary modifications/alterations
- Nuisance alarms and disabled annunciators
- Excessive noise
- Missing labels or labels oriented such that they cannot be seen or read easily
- Poor lighting
- High temperatures or high humidity (heat stress factors)
- Unusual plant or equipment conditions

- Poor accessibility, cramped conditions, or awkward layout of equipment

Administrative barriers, such as standard operating procedures or the enforcement of critical skill levels may also fail. Some of the common causes for failure of administrative barriers include:

- Two or more actions embedded in one procedural step
- Vague expectations and standards
- Superficial document reviews or the lack of a qualified reviewer process for technical procedure development
- Critical steps not identified in procedures and work packages
- Excessive work package backlog that exceeds planner resources
- Work packages planned without inclusion of operating experience
- Unresponsive procedure revision process
- Unavailable foreign material exclusion (FME) caps and covers
- Excessive deferred preventive maintenance
- Insufficient staffing leading to excessive overtime, workload, and fatigue
- Routine authorization to exceed overtime limits (leading to chronic fatigue)
- Inadequate time for direct supervision of work in the field
- Unclear qualification standards
- Incomplete or missing electrical load lists to aid in ground isolation

Pitfall 6: Failing to Identify and Minimize the Gap between Work-as-Imagined and Work-as-Done

An unhealthy culture or imbedded *latent organizational weaknesses* can degrade an organization's ability to deal with these common pitfalls (Figure 4-1). Latent organizational weaknesses are hidden deficiencies in management control processes (for example, strategy, policies, work control, training, and resource allocation) or values (shared beliefs, attitudes, norms, and assumptions). These create workplace conditions (human performance error precursors) that can lead to error and degrade the integrity of operational defenses (Reason, 1997).

The decisions and activities of managers determine what is done, how well it is done, and when it is done. Yet even the most conscientious organization has gaps between management expectations (work-as-imagined) and on-the-ground operations (work-as-done). If the organization is not mindful, managers and supervisors may fail to note these gaps. Alternatively, they may know the gap exists, but fail to take action to minimize them. Failure to continuously identify and minimize the gap between the ideal and real operations will result in practical drift and bad habits that can degrade the HRO.

A graphical representation of how organizational events and accidents occur is provided in Figure 4-4, developed by Reason (1997). This model links the various contributing elements into a coherent sequence that runs bottom-up in causation and top-down in investigation. The causal sequence begins with organizational factors like strategic decisions and organizational processes including budgeting, planning, scheduling, and managing. These processes are shaped by the *organizational culture.* In Figure 4-4, the organization overcommits its resources by promising to deliver more product than possible using its current level of operations.

The consequences of this decision create latent conditions that place stress on employees to meet the production goals. These conditions are communicated throughout the organization to local workplaces such as control rooms, work areas, and maintenance facilities, and reveal themselves as negative workplace factors. For example, the emphasis on production rate creates undue time pressure on employees and can result in poor human-machine interfaces, understaffing, poor supervisor-employee ratios, lack of maintenance, lower employee morale, and poor communication.

Within the workplace, these local workplace factors can combine with natural human performance tendencies such as limited attention,

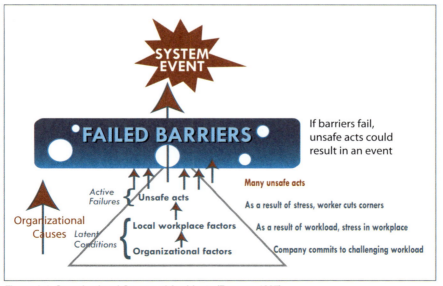

Figure 4-4. Organizational Causes of Accidents (Reason, 1997)

> ### Sharp End versus Blunt End
>
> The sharp end represents people who are in direct contact with the safety-critical process (for example, the pilot, the surgeon, or the production technician). The blunt end is the organization or set of organizations that supports and drives activities at the sharp end (for example, the pilot's airline, the surgeon's hospital administration, or the technician's regulating body). The blunt end shapes, creates, and can even encourage opportunities for errors at the sharp end.
>
> *(Dekker, 2006, p. 59)*

> ### HRO Practice 2: Reduce System Variability
>
> To reduce system variability:
>
> • Deploy the safety system (Break-the-Chain Framework).
>
> • Evaluate the operation of the safety system.
>
> • Adjust processes.

habit patterns, assumptions, complacency, or mental shortcuts. Together, these produce active errors and violations[7], which are collectively termed *unsafe acts*.

Large numbers of these unsafe acts will occur, but only a few of them will penetrate the defenses. The penetrations occur where defenses have been weakened by latent conditions. Given a large enough number or the "right" combination of barrier penetrations, a system accident can occur.

Deploy the Break-the-Chain Safety Framework

The Break-the-Chain Framework[8] was developed to provide HROs with a practical tool for dealing with the common operational pitfalls identified earlier in this chapter. The concept behind this model is simple: it is designed to interrupt the sequence of events from human error to major consequence, wherever possible and as many times as possible. The Break-the-Chain Framework consists of six steps, shown in Figure 4-5, that correlate to the common pitfalls previously discussed:

- Identify the consequence to avoid

- Identify and minimize the hazard

- Reduce human performance error precursors

- Manage the defenses

- Reduce the vulnerability of the hazard through a strong culture of reliability

- Minimize the gap between work-as-imagined and work-as-done

The Break-the-Chain Framework reinforces the activities associated with all of the HRO practices.

Chapter 4 | 97

Step 1: Identify the Consequence to Avoid
(HRO Practice 1,2)

The first step in the Break-the-Chain Framework is to focus on the last link of the chain, the consequences of the system accident that the organization is trying to prevent (Figure 4-5). The mandate to avoid these consequences originates with management's clear communication of operational safety goals.

Once the catastrophic consequences have been identified, they should be listed in priority order (i.e., with the least desirable consequence at the top). For example, an operation might list the following as consequences to avoid, beginning with the most undesirable event:

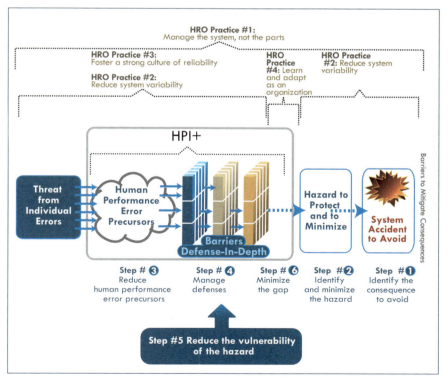

Figure 4-5. The Break-the-Chain Framework and its Relationship to the HRO Practices

1. Facility explosion

2. Radiation exposure

3. Chemical fire

4. Dispersion of hazardous chemicals

This prioritization is important for four reasons:

- It serves as an important reminder to all employees of the potential catastrophic consequences they must strive to avoid each day.

- It pinpoints where defensive barriers are most needed; as one would expect, the severity of the consequences will drive the number and type of barriers selected.

- It ensures that the defensive barriers associated with the highest priority consequences will receive top protection against degradation.

- It encourages a constant review of resources against consequences, focusing attention on making sure the most severe consequences are avoided at all times and at any cost.

This last point is critical; in a high-hazard operation, efforts to protect against catastrophic events should never be diluted by an organization's efforts to prevent less-consequential events. Focus must be maintained on system accidents to assure that the needed attention and resources are available to prevent them.

Step 2: Identify and Minimize the Hazard
(HRO Practice 1,2)

The second step in the Break-the-Chain Framework is to identify and minimize the physical hazard, while maintaining production (Figure 4-5). After identifying the hazard, there

Chapter 4 | **99**

are two approaches to minimize it. First, actions are taken to reduce the physical hazard that can be impacted by the threat. Second, attempts are made to reduce the interactive complexity and tight coupling within the operation or, conversely, to decrease the response time of the organization so an event can be recognized and responded to more quickly. The intent of these two approaches is to remove or reduce the hazard so that the consequences of an accident are minimized to the extent possible.

Identify the Hazard

The first order of business is to identify the hazards associated with the operation; in particular, to identify hazards that could lead to consequential system accidents. The second order of business is to ensure employees maintain a chronic unease regarding these identified hazards. A constant influx of energy by management is needed to overcome the natural human tendency toward complacency; as a manager, you must strive to maintain a heightened awareness and respect for operational hazards among all employees.

Minimize the Physical Hazard

To avoid the consequences identified in Step 1, the hazard must be known and understood. For example, the hazard associated with the top priority consequence, explosion of the facility, might be explosive chemicals. This hazard might be reduced by one or more of the following actions:

- Substituting less hazardous chemicals.

- Preventing energy coming in contact with explosive chemicals.

- Minimizing the stockpiling of chemicals.

- Increasing the distance between quantities of chemicals or explosives.
- Minimizing the quantity of chemicals or explosives.

Not all organizations can reduce the hazard associated with their operations. For example, nuclear reactors can't use non-nuclear materials in their reactor cores nor can they defy physics— there will always be residual heat to deal with from the decay of radioactive by-products. The important point is to give careful thought to any possible ways of minimizing the hazard and hence mitigating the consequences before dismissing them as impractical—and to make sure that a sense of complacency doesn't influence cost-risk decisions.

Reduce Interactive Complexity and Tight Coupling

A second approach to minimizing the hazard is to reduce the effects of the system's interactive complexity and tight coupling. Concern about these system characteristics originated with Perrow's study of the Three Mile Island accident (1999), which focused on the interactively-complex and tightly-coupled environment characteristic of a nuclear reactor control room. In such an environment, unplanned events can quickly escalate into an uncontrollable scenario because they occur at a pace faster than a human operator can address.

The important point about complex system interactions and tight coupling is to understand the speed of the process relative to the response time of the system (organization). No matter how slow or linear an operation is, if the ability of the system to detect and react to unanticipated changes is slower than the time for process changes to take effect, a problem exists. There

Chapter 4 | **101**

are two ways to address this problem; reduce the interactive complexity and tight coupling, or improve the response time of the organization so that process data can be collected and interpreted faster than the process unfolds. All aspects of the system (mechanical, organizational, and sociotechnical) need to be addressed to optimize response time.

Step 3: Recognize and Reduce Human Performance Error Precursors
(HRO Practice 1,2,3)

A key component of consequence avoidance is reducing the human error component that could challenge the hazard. The threat in our Break-the-Chain Framework comes from individual human errors, which occur at a rate of 4–5 errors an hour. Human error is indicated in Figure 4-5 by a large number of arrows that enter the white cloud, which represents the human error component of the Break-the-Chain Framework. The chain of events that occur here can, and must, be interrupted to avoid the undesired consequence.

To this end, we've incorporated the Human Performance Improvement (HPI) program developed by the Institute of Nuclear Power Operations (INPO) into the Break-the-Chain Framework. Much of the material presented in Steps 3 through 4 is summarized from *Human Performance Fundamentals* (INPO, 2002, 2006) and from the *Causal Analysis Handbook* (TXU, 2005) and is used with their permission. We have also added an additional step, Step 6, to explicitly evaluate the gap between work-as-imagined by the manager and work-as-done by the employee (Dekker, 2006). This feedback provides critical information about the health of the culture and the effectiveness of HRO practices. To denote this adaptation of the INPO program, the

Active Errors

The initiating action is an action by an individual, either correct, in error, or in violation, that results in a facility event. An error is an action that unintentionally departs from an expected behavior. A violation is a deliberate, intentional act to evade a known policy or procedure requirement. Active errors are those errors that have immediate, observable, undesirable outcomes in the physical facility. They can be either acts of commission or omission. The majority of initiating actions are active errors. Therefore, a strategic approach to preventing events should be the anticipation and prevention of active errors.

(U.S. DOE, 2007)

notation "HPI+" is used in this text and in Figure 4-5. The primary emphasis of HPI+ is to break the linkages between an event and the set-up factors; this preemptive break in the chain reduces the probability of a system event or accident by reducing the number of challenges on the plant's hazards from the active errors of humans. A strategic approach to preventing events will include the anticipation and prevention of active errors. The pre-existing conditions at the job site that increase the likelihood of human error during a specific action (the human performance error precursors) must be reduced.

An error-likely situation typically exists when the demands of the task exceed the capabilities of the individual performing the task, or when work conditions aggravate the limitations of human nature (Reason, 1998). To reduce the imbalance between human capabilities and environmental stressors, the human performance error mode that characterizes the situation should be determined. These error modes were described earlier in this chapter (Pitfall 3). An understanding of the applicable error mode helps both the manager and the employee take preventive action.

Next, the human performance error precursors must be identified. This is accomplished by performing a TWIN Analysis, which focuses on task demands, work environment, individual capabilities, and human nature as the four types of human error precursors. Figure 4-6 shows a sample TWIN Analysis Matrix with examples of human performance error precursors. These errors should be identified in daily pre-job briefings or other efforts made to minimize their impact on operations before work is begun.

Reducing error-likely situations reduces the probability of accidents by maintaining *positive control*, a term used to indicate that "what happens is what was intended to happen and is all that happens." (INPO, 2006)). Positive control reduces the number of challenges on the defenses.

Step 4: Manage the Defenses (HRO Practice 1,2,3) Another part of the HPI+ portion of the Break-the-Chain Framework, this step focuses on ensuring that the defense barriers are adequate to prevent or mitigate the consequences of a system accident (Figure 4-5). The type and number of barriers and the level of effort needed to protect them are dictated by the level of consequence and the type of hazard associated with the operation.

Defense-in-depth is achieved by embedding overlapping defenses into the organization, its culture, and the physical facility. Thus, if one defense fails or is ineffective, other systematically-placed redundant defenses will fulfill the same defensive function. The two primary lines of defense—engineered and administrative defenses—work together to anticipate, prevent, or mitigate active errors and thus prevent a system accident.

Engineered defenses or controls are designed into the system and include hardware, software, and equipment that affect people's behavior, choices, and attitudes. Engineered controls can be active or passive. Active controls are typically equipment such as pumps or valves that perform a specific safety-related function. Passive controls include pipes, vessels, and earthen berms that provide containment and generally do not have moving parts.

Administrative defenses, such as procedures, inform people about what to do, when to do it, where to do it, and how well to do it, and are usually documented in various written policies,

> **HPI+ Aims To Prevent System Accidents (But May Do More)**
>
> As used in this guide, the HPI+ process of the Break-the-Chain Framework (Steps 3 through 6) is meant to prevent or mitigate the system accident, not to reduce individual accidents.
>
> A fortuitous by-product of the process, however, may be increased industrial safety—that is, fewer individual accidents—and thus a decrease in lost time due to accidents and the number of reportable injuries.

Task Demands	Individual Capabilities
Interpretation Requirements	Schedule Pressure to Get the Work Done
High Workload (Memory Requirements)	First Time Task
Simultaneous—Multiple Tasks	Knowingly Broke a Rule
Unexpected Conditions Encountered	Problem Solved Incorrectly (inaccurate mental model)
Time Pressure	Fatigue or Illness
Repetitive Actions/Monotony	Lack of Experience With Tasks
Unclear Goals, Roles, or Responsibilities	Inaccurate Mental Model of Tasks
Lack of or Unclear Standards	Misunderstood Communication
Confusing Procedure/Vague Guidance	No Communication
Delays, Idle Time, Employee Got Lost	Personal Issue—Lost Focus (medical, financial emotional)

Work Environment	Human Nature
Confusing Controls/Display	Made Bad Assumption
Over Confidence	Mind Set (I could have sworn it was right)
Distractions/Interruptions	Complacency (task done many times before)
Unexpected Equipment Condition	Disoriented or Confused During a Task
Production Emphasis by Supervisors	Mental Shortcut (assumptions easily confirmed)
Unavailable Parts or Tools—Made Do	Boring Task
Changes/Departure from Routine	Work with People I do not Know or Like
Personality Conflicts	On the Job Stress (perceived threat to well-being)
Work-Arounds	Habit Patterns Caused by Wrong Actions Left Unchecked for Long Time
Hidden Systems Response	Inaccurate Risk or Hazard Perception
Adverse Environmental Condition (heat/cold)	Focused on Task—Missed Big Picture
Poor Acccess to Equipment/Human Factors	Limited Short-Term Memory
Swing Shift Work	Uncertain About Job Requirements

Figure 4-6. TWIN Analysis Matrix (TXU, 2005)

Chapter 4 | 105

programs, and plans. Administrative controls rely on human judgment, training, and personal initiative to follow the direction contained in documents.

As might be expected, some controls are more reliable than others. In general, physical defenses tend to perform their intended functions despite human action or inaction. Engineered controls, such as physical interlocks and equipment design, are more reliable than administrative controls which depend on people to follow them, such as procedures, human performance tools, and training programs. The most reliable engineered defenses are passive (e.g., pipes, vessels, and berms) because they require little to no operational or maintenance support to remain effective, and thus are not dependent on a significant amount of human involvement. If the effectiveness of a defense mechanism relies on human performance (e.g., procedures, training, self-checking, and verification) it is less reliable. If operational safety and reliability are dependent on human performance during risk-important activities, the physical hazard is more vulnerable to human errors. Reliability is related to the dependability of the defense or barrier to perform its intended function when needed. If it is imperative to prevent error, then physical, engineered controls are more appropriate.

There are two applications of defenses: defenses to reduce the probability of a system accident and defenses to mitigate the consequences of a system accident (reduces the impact on employees, the environment, and the local community).

Manage Defenses to Reduce the Probability of the System Accident
The first part of managing defenses is to reduce the vulnerability of the hazard to human

error, and thus reduce the probability of a system accident. This involves placing multiple independent barriers within the operating system to protect the hazard from the threat (Figure 4-5).

Defenses cannot be managed if they are transparent to the workforce. It is critical that planners, employees, and supervisors explicitly identify and validate the barriers, and verify their independence from each other, before work begins.

Manage Defenses to Reduce the Consequences of the System Accident

The second part of managing defenses is to mitigate the consequences of the system accident once something goes (badly) wrong. This requires multiple independent barriers that act as buffers to lessen the impact of an accident (Figure 4-5). The type and number of barriers to mitigate the effects of an event and the level of effort to protect them are dictated by the type of hazard and probable consequences. These barriers are the final defenses between the hazard and total catastrophe. Typically, they are structural barriers designed to contain the effects of explosions (or prevent propagation) and to prevent chemical or radiological releases.

Step 5: Reduce Vulnerability of the Hazard Through a Strong Culture of Reliability

(HRO Practice 1,2,3)

Steps 1 through 4 of the Break-the-Chain Framework make the operational hazard less vulnerable to human error. To execute these steps successfully and consistently, day in and day out, without observable signs of significant events, requires an army of trained and experienced personnel who conscientiously follow the established HRO practices. The foot soldiers in this army must maintain their proficiency through continuous hands-on work. They must be trained and socialized so they can make judgment calls on the shop floor that will reflect the shared HRO values. They must have the authority to make time-critical decisions when situations require this action. In a nutshell, they must be part of an organization that has a strong culture of reliability.

Decentralized authority gives employees the authority to make time-critical decisions on the shop floor, but this alone is not enough to ensure that the decisions will be appropriate from a safety and reliability perspective. To ensure this additional quality and safety requires a supportive infrastructure that allows employees to maintain positive control (INPO, 2006). It is critical that all employees have extensive training on the technical aspects of the safety measures and on the HRO practices, as well as continuous hands-on training on the specific systems they operate.

A culture of reliability provides consistent demonstration of conservative operational decisions. To develop this consistency, employees must be empowered to openly identify issues. Issues must be promptly and effectively resolved so they do not continue to plague the work force or work flow, and lessons must be openly shared so that the entire organization can learn from them. In addition, a hands-on approach to job skills ensures that employees stay proficient with all tasks and thus reduce errors incurred during the start up of new processes. The attributes of a strong culture of reliability are further discussed in Chapter 5.

Step 6: Minimize the Gap between Work-as-Imagined and Work-as-Done

(HRO Practice 1,4)

Gaps between work-as-imagined by the manager and work-as-done by the employee exist in every operation (Figure 4-5). The fact that these gaps exist is not the concern. The problem occurs when the organization is unaware of the gaps or does not know the magnitude or extent of the gaps across the operation. Failure to identify and quantify gaps between the ideal and the real makes it impossible for managers to monitor the health of the HRO and evaluate the effectiveness of corrective actions. To remedy this, the HPI+ process places special emphasis on evaluating and closing the gap between work-as-imagined and work-as-done.

Minimizing the gap between work-as-imagined and work-as-done requires a multi-tiered approach. The first tier (Tier 0) involves management actions to ensure that the critical components of the safety system (Break-the-Chain Framework) are in place before work is begun. These components include both the various controls and the verification measures needed to ensure that these controls are functional and independent.

Next (Tier 1), managers need to stress the importance of continuous supervisor-employee feedback that focuses on identifying gaps between the ideal (work-as-imagined) and the actual (work-as-done). This feedback allows human performance error precursors and flawed barriers to be identified quickly. When these error-likely situations are discovered, work must be stopped until the situations are addressed; otherwise errors may be compounded.

Chapter 4   **109**

The next tier (Tier 2) includes making a high-level scan of operations by tracking operational data and using it to identify trends that indicate repeat occurrences or event precursors. Data should be mined to reveal hidden events that are not otherwise evident. Such data analyses will allow managers to undertake detailed investigations and take corrective actions before problems escalate.

Low-consequence system events also provide insight into systemic problems (Tier 3). These events should be viewed as information-rich opportunities that can highlight significant gaps between work-as-imagined versus work-as-done or indicate the existence of a type of error that is not covered by the current system design. The significance of these events lies not in their actual consequences but in their potential consequences. In other words, some of these events might have had grave consequences, had not luck intervened.

The final tier in Step 6 (Tier 4) involves learning from other high-hazard operations. This includes studying and learning from others' misfortunes (i.e., lessons learned from external accident investigations) as well as adapting and benchmarking best business practices from similar industries.

The tiered approach to organizational learning is described in more detail in Chapter 6.

Illustrative Examples: Applying the Break-the-Chain Framework

The following two examples are provided to help you better visualize the use of the Break-the-Chain Framework in everyday operations. In the first example, the framework is applied to a situation in which the organization wants to avoid the consequences of an individual accident (although the Break-the-Chain Framework was developed to prevent system accidents, it can also be applied to industrial accidents). The second example summarizes the steps used to prevent a system accident at a facility that uses explosive chemicals.

Example 1: Industrial safety example to prevent individual accidents

Situation: Snow and ice present a hazard for plant employees.

- *Step 1: Identify the consequence to avoid.* The company wants to prevent individuals from slipping and falling, which could result in injuries (consequences) such as broken hips or other bones.

- *Step 2: Identify and minimize the hazard.* The hazard is snow and ice. The hazard is minimized through the use of an ice-preventing agent before the snow begins, and by plowing and using ice melt after the snow has fallen and ice has formed. Even if the ice is not totally removed, the hazard will at least be reduced.

- *Step 3: Reduce human performance error precursors.* The employees are made aware of the upcoming bad weather (the error-likely situation) by a loudspeaker announcement. A warning about possible snow and ice and the need for care to prevent falls and associated injuries is included and the employees are urged to wear appropriate footwear to work on the following day (e.g., soft sole shoes or ice grippers).

- *Step 4: Manage the defenses.* The employees think about and take action to implement

Chapter 4 | **111**

defensive barriers to avoid slipping. Actions could include wearing footwear with soft rubber soles, parking in areas where there is no ice, or calling the plant shuttle to avoid having to walk across the parking lot. The final barrier used to prevent a fall would be to avoid walking on any visible ice. Further measures such as wearing knee or hip pads could be taken to mitigate the consequences of a fall.

- *Step 5: Reduce vulnerability of the hazard through a strong culture of reliability.* The more people walk on the ice, the higher the likelihood that a slip will occur. Therefore, the organization must continually instill in each employee the necessity of following Steps 1 through 4 (i.e., instill a culture of reliability). Each employee, when faced with a choice (e.g., to walk across the parking lot or call a shuttle), must be trained to make the right decision.

- *Step 6: Minimize gap between the ideal (work-as-imagined) and the real (work-as-done).* To ensure that employees follow safety directives, the organization can post safety personnel in the parking lot to remind employees of the hazard and to ensure that barriers (e.g., shoes, shuttle, and avoidance of icy areas) are used. If an accident does occur, feedback about the accident and corrective actions to preclude future similar events should be immediate.

Example 2: Fire safety example to avoid system accident

Situation: Facility fires resulting in death and release of toxic fumes.

- *Step 1: Identify consequence to avoid.* The type of accident the operation needs to avoid is a facility fire. Consequences of such a fire could involve death and injury to personnel and bystanders, destruction of the facility and other property, and socioeconomic impacts to the community.

- *Step 2: Identify and minimize the hazard.* The hazard to remove or restrict is the amount of combustible material that can be taken into work areas. This will minimize the potential for large facility heat loadings on the structure and its contents.

- *Step 3: Reduce human performance error precursors.* The organization must first make the employees aware of error-likely situations that could result in too many combustibles in the work area. All employees must have access to and review a list of prohibited articles and actions on a routine basis.

- *Step 4: Manage the defenses.* The defenses to prevent or minimize the facility fire include establishing and following combustible-loading procedures, training employees, checking employees who enter work areas for combustibles, and ensuring fire detection and fire suppression systems are functional on a daily basis.

- *Step 5: Reduce vulnerability of the hazard through a strong culture of reliability.* The greater the amount of combustible-loading at the facility, the higher the likelihood of a consequential fire. Therefore, the organization must continually instill in each employee the necessity of following Steps 1 through 4. The employees must understand the importance of following the procedures and ensuring that combustibles are kept to a minimum; this is instilled through a strong culture of reliability. Each employee, when faced

Chapter 4 | **113**

with a choice such as whether to follow the combustible-loading requirements or to work around those requirements to save time, must be trained to make the right call.

- *Step 6: Minimize gap between the ideal (work-as-imagined) and the real (work-as-done).* Each day before work is begun, supervisors should review the error-likely situations with employees, explicitly call out the various barriers that should be in place, and verify with employees that these barriers are actually in place. These pre-work meetings should be used to instill a sense of teamwork and encourage all employees to identify and address any latent organizational weaknesses or signs of an unhealthy culture.

Evaluate the Operation of the Safety System

Your work as a manager does not stop once you have implemented an HRO safety system appropriate for your organization. To sustain high reliability operations, you must continually evaluate and refine the operation of various processes within the system. Negative trends, such as an increase in variability from the established safety system, indicate a greater likelihood of a system accident.

Systematically Adjust Processes

To identify and analyze trends, data should be collected and tracked over a long enough period to develop a rate, or frequency of occurrence of variation from the safety system, for each process. Once a rate has been established, use statistical tools to determine the process capability and evaluate whether it is adequately controlled; Lean manufacturing tools can identify and eliminate sources of wasted efforts and Six Sigma tools can identify and minimize sources of variation from the established safety processes. These processes can be applied to mechanical operating or production systems as well as to administrative systems. Applying both of these tools to selected production processes will reduce variability of the safety system over time, thereby improving the reliability of the operation.

Evaluation of the various system processes will allow you to adjust processes. For each problem area you discover, you should implement corrective actions, incorporate information from lessons learned, and continue to evaluate and refine the system processes.

Implement Effective Corrective Actions

Corrective actions (Corcoran, 2007b) identified to address weaknesses in the system (as evidenced by system events) should aim to:

- Fix the problem.
- Fix the process that created the problem.
- Fix every process that should have detected the problem or its causal factors before the event.

Corrective actions are required for each causal factor, each identified human performance error precursor, and each flawed barrier. They are also required for those factors known as extraneous conditions adverse to quality (ECAQ) which, although they did not contribute to the event in question, are found to be flawed and require correction. Depending on the pervasiveness of the causal factors across the organization, the corrective actions may be modified to apply to the entire organization or may be applied immediately to specific processes or departments.

There are four basic types of corrective actions, differentiated by their relationship to the stated problem:

Corrective Actions
All too often corrective actions are the Achilles' heel of an organization working to become an HRO. Effective corrective actions are difficult to develop and implement; consequently, managers often implement corrective actions that fail to address the root of the problem.

- Accommodational
- Ceremonial or political
- Symptomatic
- Fundamental

Although each of the four types may be appropriate under specific circumstances, only the fundamental type actually corrects the root cause of the system problem. When used inappropriately or exclusively, the other types of corrective actions may actually do more harm than good. See if any of the following descriptions bring back bad memories of situations that have occurred in your organization.

Accommodational corrective actions address the problem by (1) changing the norm, requirement, or expectation that makes the condition a problem or (2) changing the system, so that the condition is no longer a problem.

Accommodational corrective actions include:

- Canceling school rather than removing snow promptly.
- Getting a technical specification change or regulatory exemption because it is inconvenient to meet the existing technical specification or requirement.

Some interim compensatory measures are accommodating; for example, one might accommodate a gasoline leak in the joint between the tank and the fill pipe by the interim compensatory measure of only filling the tank part way.

Accommodational corrective actions can easily send the wrong message to lower level employees, even when the action is the best approach under the circumstances. This tendency can be

> **Lower Your Expectations?**
>
> The archetypical accommodational corrective action is captured by the humorous poster sometimes seen in diners: "If our service does not meet your expectations, please lower your expectations."
>
> *(Corcoran, 2007a)*

overcome if managers take the time to explain to the relevant work groups what corrective actions are being taken and why these are appropriate.

Ceremonial or *political corrective actions* invoke tradition, ritual, publicity, or gatherings to address problems even when these actions have no factually established causal relationship with the problem at hand. Such actions may have their purpose, but they should not be expected to have measurable impacts on the frequency or severity of future problems of similar types. These actions may include:

- Lengthy reports
- Bulletins and news sheets
- Attempts to influence employee behavior without an attempt to change management behavior
- Pass-around reading that does not clearly capture the behavior changes required
- Warnings and other postings that are not effectively located or are not relevant to employees' activities

These seemingly ineffective actions tend to disillusion employees. Admit it—haven't you rolled your eyes and muttered, "Here we go again," at least once in your career in response to this type of corrective action?

Symptomatic corrective actions address the symptoms of the stated problem without addressing the underlying causes. They often result in fire drills that mobilize the organization to work on the symptom du jour. Such actions, which can be crucial to operations, may include the following:

- Putting out real fires
- Fixing broken machinery

Chapter 4 | **117**

- Providing medical attention to injured employees

Many organizations have elaborate systems for rapid deployment of symptomatic corrective actions. Sometimes this is because the basic nature of the industrial process requires this type of immediate response, sometimes it is to provide defenses-in-depth, and sometimes it is because the organization has not learned the value of fundamental corrective actions.

The routine corrective actions reported to regulatory authorities in response to inspection findings and reportable occurrences are often symptomatic actions. These actions provide an apparent responsiveness to the condition, and they can be audited.

To address the basic fundamental underlying causes of the problem at hand, *fundamental corrective actions* are required. These actions "drive a stake through the heart of the problem." The difficulty is that to determine appropriate fundamental corrective actions, it is almost always necessary to undertake a thoughtful and objective analysis of how and why the problems occurred. Fundamental corrective actions can include:

- Replacing dysfunctional managers
- Changing the organizational culture
- Changing dysfunctional processes

Human error is inextricably connected to features of the tasks and tools that people work with, and to the features of the work environment. Human errors represent the leakage that occurs around the edges of an organization when you put pressure on the system without considering other factors. It is important to consider both the system and the culture when recommending corrective actions to ensure that such actions truly are effective for the specific organization and system.

Human error is a consequence. Efforts to understand human error should ultimately point to changes that will remove the error potential from the organizational system. To be effective, corrective actions must be SMART (specific, measurable, agreed-to, realistic, and time-bound). Corrective actions can range from easy, but often ineffective, low-end actions (for example, retraining, demoting or getting rid of the bad apple, or tightening procedures) to high-end actions (for example, structural decisions regarding resources, workplace technologies, and pressures) (Dekker, 2006).

High-end fixes are difficult, expensive, time-consuming, and cut across divisional lines. The ability of managers to embrace high-end countermeasures hinges on whether these corrective actions make sense to them in the context of their goals, knowledge, and focus of attention. Low-end fixes such as retraining or reprimanding employees, writing new procedures, and adding a bit more technology typically do not address the conditions that may produce errors. As Dekker (2006, p.183) says, "Your human error problem is an organizational problem. Your human error problem is as complex as the organization that helped create it." Thus, it is important to resist the urge to use common or ineffective quick fixes. Instead, you should strive to understand and address the true causes of the problem.

Learn Lessons

As we all know, learning is hard—especially for those with closed minds. Whereas corrective actions are meant to address specific system or process problems, lessons to be learned (LTBL) are meant to result in an observed behavior change. They reflect organizational changes in thinking and behavior that result from the event investigation. Lessons to be learned are developed for those things for which specific corrective actions cannot remedy. For example, a corrective action may include modifying a procedure to ensure that it produces the desired result. The associated lesson to be learned may involve encouraging employees to actually use the modified procedure in their daily work by providing the rationale behind its use.

As adopted from William Corcoran's *Phoenix Handbook*, the term *lessons to be learned* is different from *lessons learned*. Lessons to be learned become lessons learned only after they have been:

- Read and understood
- Internalized
- Acted upon
- Verified effective (i.e., they have modified the behavior of the target group)

This typically requires establishing proof of behavior modification. For example, verification may entail measuring the effectiveness of retraining efforts by testing employees whose behaviors were supposed to be changed after a specified period of time (e.g., six months or one year). If the employees' behavior is modified to incorporate the principles of the LTBL, verification is complete.

Verify Corrective Measures Provide Desired Change

The steps to develop and implement corrective actions parallel those to develop and implement strategy. First, you must identify what needs to be corrected, and then you must establish the measures, assign a target or targets, and develop initiatives to implement the corrective actions. The key, however, is to track how well the corrective actions address the identified problem and to make any necessary adjustments—otherwise there is no organizational learning.

To ensure corrective actions truly are addressing the intended problems, independent evaluations should be made to determine the degree of desired behavior modification attained, the degree to which corrective actions have been implemented, the effectiveness of the corrective actions, and any detrimental impacts they may have inadvertently caused.

Chapter 5

Chapter 5

Fostering a Culture of Reliability

This chapter answers the following questions:

- Why is organizational culture important to an HRO?

- What is the difference between a safety culture and a culture of reliability?

- Why does my HRO organization need to foster a culture of reliability?

- How do I, as a manager, foster a culture of reliability?

Our contention in this guide is that an organization must assimilate the four HRO practices presented in Chapter 1 and discussed in more detail in Chapters 4–6 to ensure high reliability operations. A healthy safety culture— what we call a culture of reliability—is critical to such assimilation. Organizations with a culture of reliability are characterized by communications founded on mutual trust, by shared perceptions of the importance of safety, and by confidence in the efficacy of preventive measures (Booth in ACSNI, 1993). To establish this level of trust requires active management involvement at every level—from the shop floor to the senior managers' offices.

This chapter, which focuses on HRO Practice 3, Foster a Culture of Reliability, is divided into two sections. The first explains what we mean by a culture of reliability as a frame of reference for understanding this concept as it relates to an

HRO. The second section provides a step-by-step approach to help you, as a manager, develop the strong culture of reliability needed to achieve and sustain high reliability operations.

What is a Culture of Reliability?

We first introduced the concepts of safety culture and culture of reliability in Chapter 2. This chapter provides a more in-depth explanation of each of these terms. In essence, a culture of reliability is a safety culture that manifests the positive characteristics necessary for high reliability operations. A culture of reliability is needed to ensure that the intent of the HRO practices is maintained; it provides the stamina an organization needs to sustain the HRO practices. Continual evaluation of the culture is needed to determine the effectiveness of the HRO practices being internalized and implemented by the employees. For example, if you observe an unsafe act on the shop floor, you can be pretty sure that it reflects the accepted safety culture of the organization. Employee behavior reflects the work environment; thus, it is unlikely that such an act is an anomaly. In this respect, the information obtained from event investigations, if properly characterized and evaluated, can be used as an indicator of the health of the culture of the organization. The evaluation of culture as a means of evaluating the effectiveness of an organization's HRO practices is discussed in more detail in Chapter 7.

The Basics of Organizational Culture

The concept of safety culture is an outgrowth of the concept of organizational culture, a term generally credited to Dr. Edgar Schein (1992). Organizational culture is to the organization as personality and character are to the individual. As

---

HRO Practice 3: Foster a Strong Culture of Reliability

A strong culture of reliability requires that managers:

- Provide the capability and the expectation to make conservative decisions.
- Retain proficiency through continuous hands-on work.
- Provide the ability to openly question and verify safety and demonstrate a culture of reliability.

organizations grow and succeed, they undergo the same kind of learning process as individuals. The beliefs and values of the group's founders and leaders gradually become shared values that are taken for granted as long as the organization is successful in fulfilling its mission and managing itself internally. It is the past history of success that strengthens and solidifies cultural beliefs and values. Schein suggests that organizational culture has three layers: artifacts, espoused beliefs and values, and the deeper underlying assumptions (Figure 5-1 on the following page).

Schein's organizational model illuminates culture from the standpoint of the observer. As shown in Figure 5-1, the first and most cursory level represents *artifacts* (organizational attributes) which can be seen, felt, and heard by the uninitiated observer. These include the organization's facilities, offices, furnishings, and visible awards and recognition; the way its members dress; and how members visibly interact with each other and with outsiders (U.S. DOE, 2007).

The next level deals with the *espoused beliefs and values* (professed culture) of the organization's members. Company slogans, mission statements, and other operational creeds may express these espoused values, and local and personal values within the organization are likely to reflect those espoused by the organization. The professed culture can be determined through interviews of the organization's membership, the use of questionnaires, and reviews of employee behavior obtained from investigative tools such as Causal Factors Analysis (CFA).

The third and deepest level of the organization is its underlying assumptions. These cultural

---

Organizational Culture

- We are constantly surrounded by culture; it is enacted and created through our interactions with others.

- Managers can use culture to better understand the dynamics of organizational change.

- To effect evolutionary change within an organization, its leaders must first understand the dynamics of culture.

(Schein, 2007)

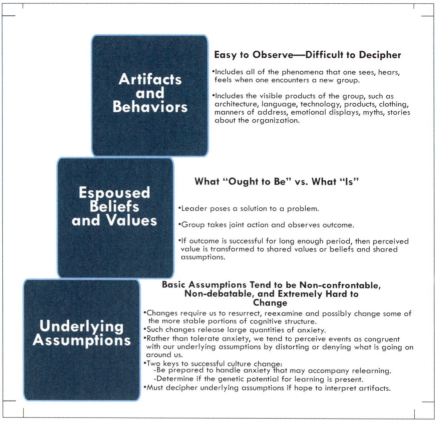

Figure 5-1. Schein Levels of Culture (Schein, 1992)

elements are unseen and not cognitively identified in everyday interactions between organizational members. Frequently, any discussion of these elements within the organization is taboo, and many of these unspoken rules exist without the conscious knowledge of the membership. Members with sufficient longevity to understand this deepest level of organizational culture usually become acclimatized to the unspoken assumptions over time, thus reinforcing their invisibility.

Chapter 5 | 125

Because the elements of culture are learned intuitively by members of the organization, changes in culture require much discussion, communication, and learning, and take a long time to bring to fruition. Likewise, changing behaviors is also difficult because people have very strong patterns that they follow from habit.

In summary, an organization's culture is best defined by the shared basic assumptions that it has developed over time. Culture is the sum total of the organization's learning. **The culture of a group can be defined as a pattern of shared basic assumptions, learned by the group as it solved its problems of external adaptation and internal integration, that has worked well enough to be considered valid and, therefore, is taught to new members as the correct way to perceive, think, and feel in relation to those problems.** In short, culture is "the way we do things around here."

Safety Culture (U.S. DOE, 2007)

Safety culture is that portion of a company's organizational culture that relates to operational and system safety. Employees that become too complacent about the technology and the fact that "there hasn't been a major event here" may share beliefs about safety that are detrimental to high reliability operations. Such employees may come to believe, usually unconsciously, that their facility or system is robust and has a comfortable safety margin. This mindset can be very dangerous.

In contrast, if the organization cultivates and maintains a culture of reliability, employees will exhibit chronic unease about operations and continually question the validity of the safety system with respect to its ability to preclude a catastrophic accident. Such constant vigilance is

---

Watch Your Safety Culture

Company Omega is a high-hazard operation with a good safety record and corresponding safety culture that strongly supports the idea that its operational system is robust. This collective assumption, a normal response to good safety statistics, weakens the employees' sense of urgency about repairing defective equipment; as a result, one of the system's physical barriers fails. Because the plant is robust, operators don't follow all the procedures; as a result this administrative barrier fails. Also because the plant is robust, employees fail to report minor problems or unusual observations, thus the organization fails to learn about problems in the system and take appropriate corrective actions. Finally, because the plant is robust, an operator makes a nonconservative decision in a situation of uncertainty, causing the "last chance" barrier to fail. The outcome is a system accident that kills employees and members of the community, and causes the facility to be permanently closed.

> **The Importance Of Organizational Culture**
>
> Part of the effectiveness of organizations lies in the way in which they are able to bring together large numbers of people and imbue them for a sufficient time with sufficient similarity of approach, outlook, and priorities to enable them to achieve collective, sustained responses which would be impossible if a group of unorganized individuals were to face the same problem. However, this very property also brings with it the dangers of a collective blindness to important issues; the danger that some vital factors may be left outside the bounds of the organizational perception."
>
> *(Turner and Pidgeon, 1997)*

difficult and defies human nature, but is essential for an HRO.

How to Foster a Strong Culture of Reliability

An important component to the success of an HRO is the ability to decentralize decision making related to safety issues to those closest to the problem. Such decentralization permits rapid yet appropriate responses to dangers (i.e., enables operators to contain the unexpected). It requires however a culture of reliability, such that safety measures deemed important to avoid the system accident (e.g., formal rules and standard operating procedures) are reliably followed and all deviations from the safety system are represented by conservative decisions.

A culture of reliability starts with you, the manager. As Deming stated (1994), to achieve the desired result, a leader of transformation must learn and understand not only the psychology of individuals, but that of groups. It is your job to ensure that employees buy into the safety system, police the safety system, and learn to make operational decisions that stay within the safety envelope established by the safety system.

Enable Employees to Make Conservative Decisions

If you expect your employees to make consistently conservative, appropriate decisions about operational safety, it is your job to make sure they have a strong safety and operational foundation and a supportive infrastructure to help them maintain positive control (INPO, 2006) of their work processes once the decisions are made.

Training and education are essential components for a prepared workforce. Continuous hands-on training related to equipment and safety systems provides staff with the proficiency to ensure their decisions are grounded in the challenges of real-life physical processes. Technical education ensures that employees understand the fundamental underpinnings of the technical systems that they use each day. It also provides them with knowledge about safety culture, organizational learning, and conservative decision making that enables them to make contextual decisions that reflect your safety expectations.

To support your employees in making such decisions, you must provide a robust infrastructure that encompasses engineering support, tooling support, and maintenance of critical safety systems. This infrastructure is needed for employees to maintain positive control (INPO, 2006) of their work environment and prevent the escalation of minor events into accidents with major consequences. An essential component of this support infrastructure is the built-in flexibility to allow rapid, decentralized decision making when the need arises. This is where your understanding of your employees, how they will react under given circumstances, and how they react with the management system is vital. This understanding is vital to ensure the proper level of autonomy for rapid decision making when unexpected events occur.

Ensure Proficiency Through Hands-On Work

There is no substitute for reality-based experience. When time-critical safety or operational decisions are required, you don't want your employees breaking out procedures for the first time. This would be like an airline pilot whose plane just lost an engine, opening up the users' manual to see what to do next, as opposed to making real-time decisions to save the passengers. Real-time safety decisions should be made by people who

Training Versus Education

Training provides the "what." It prepares the receiver to optimize the space inside the box. Training is very effective as long as things go according to plan.

Education provides an understanding of the "why" behind the "what." It allows the receiver to not only optimize the space in the box, but to recognize and adapt to the unexpected by exploiting the endless bounds outside the box.

"Therefore the leader's role is to align organizational processes and values to optimize both production and safety at the job site."

(U.S DOE, 2007, p. 4–7)

are experts, who know their processes, their equipment, and their safety systems inside and out, and who have "been-there, done-that."

Expert levels of proficiency in dealing with hazardous processes and materials can only be obtained through continuous, hands-on work experience. This requires production systems that are up and running most of the time, not down due to maintenance backlogs, long waits for raw materials, or other operational problems. As a manager, you must emphasize the continual use of process improvement tools to optimize system availability. Lean manufacturing, Six Sigma, and other tools can help you increase uptime and reduce cycle time. This will enable employees to do what they do best, work continuously to maintain their proficiency while producing product.

Of course, one could argue that, because real-time safety decisions require proficient employees, no hazardous process should ever be started before full process proficiency is demonstrated. The process of verifying start up before hazardous operations commence is discussed in more detail in Chapter 6.

Encourage Open Questioning of and Challenges to the Safety System

No safety system in the world is perfect. The viability of any safety system hinges not only on proper design, but also reflects how well it is monitored, challenged, and improved by its capable and proficient workforce.

As a manager, you want your employees to challenge the safety system. Encourage them to stop work and ask for clarification when directions are unclear. Push them toward a chronic unease with regard to safety issues; after all, they will pay the full price of a mistake that leads to a catastrophic system accident. Demand that your employees challenge the system and openly identify problems.

You must also meet the challenges of a culture of reliability; you must walk the talk, listen to the concerns of your staff, and implement actions to correct the weaknesses of the safety system and provide the level of safety required to prevent the catastrophic accident. To best accomplish this, you must spend time on the shop floor to engage your employees and root out their concerns. You must insist that employees verify for themselves the effectiveness of the safety system every day, before every job begins, without fail. The best safety measure is the questioning attitude of the concerned employee and a manager who walks the talk.

Initial verification isn't enough. Everyone— employees and managers—must police the operation of the system to ensure all procedures and safety measures are adhered to religiously. Line supervisors, who are closest to the point in the system where active errors occur, must continually provide feedback to their staff about shop floor decisions. Such immediate feedback will keep errors to a minimum (in both numbers and severity) and enable the system to operate safely and remain resilient.

Monitor, Evaluate, and Use Feedback to Recharge Your Efforts

Schein's model (Figure 5-1) representing the three levels of organizational culture probably resonates to experiences and observations you have made within your organization. Understanding these levels and how they affect the behavior of individuals and groups within an organization will help you enable your organization to learn and adapt (Chapter 6). It will also help you evaluate the effectiveness of your organization's culture with respect to the four HRO practices.

A healthy safety culture—that is, a culture of reliability—requires alignment of all three of the layers of cultural elements. In other words, the outward actions of employees regarding safety and reliability issues should match both the espoused beliefs of the organization and its deeper, underlying assumptions. Do you have a culture of reliability that will help you, as a manager, to sustain the energy-intensive efforts needed to become an HRO and then to sustain high reliability operations? If not, you need to revamp your efforts to ensure that the behavior of your organization and employees becomes better aligned with the values that you, as an HRO manager, espouse.

Chapter 6

Chapter 6

Learning and Adapting as an Organization: The Feedback Loop

This chapter answers the following questions:

- As a manager, how do I generate decision-making information?

- What sort of feedback is associated with each of the five tiers of generating organizational learning?

- How do I manage to ensure that feedback about the safety system is appropriately interpreted and integrated into day-to-day operations?

- How do I use feedback to refine the HRO safety system?

No system is perfect, no matter how well designed, and even the best-designed system is sometimes plagued by operational problems. To attain the level of operational reliability and safety needed to prevent a system accident, employees must continually improve their skill and performance levels. HRO Practice 4 focuses on organizational learning and adapting in the context of increasing the safety and reliability of the organization. This practice is essential to the HRO to ensure the safety system is constantly evaluated and refined. In this chapter, we discuss two aspects of HRO Practice 4, those actions needed to generate feedback for well-informed decision making, and how to integrate and interpret this feedback to enable better decision-

> **Management In Any Form Is Prediction**
> Managers predict future outcomes, with the risk of being wrong, based on observations of the past. Rational prediction builds knowledge through systematic revision and extension of theoretical principles; such a revision is based on a comparison of prediction and observation. Without theory, there is no learning.
>
> *Deming, 1994)*

High Reliability Operations • A Practical Guide to Avoid the System Accident

making. Then we discuss how to use feedback and other system approaches to reduce variability.

In Chapter 4, we discussed how feedback is used to make decisions (Step 6 of the Break-the-Chain Framework). In this chapter, we introduce a five-tiered approach to obtaining feedback and information that will help you and your organization make appropriate decisions throughout all phases of operation, from start up to daily operations to routine monitoring to investigating and correcting system problems discovered in system events. These five, interrelated tiers used to gather and process information are as follows:

HRO Practice 4: Learn And Adapt As An Organization

This practice focuses on an organization's ability to use feedback to:

- Generate decision-making information.

- Refine the HRO system (reduce variability).

- *Tier 0* involves the start up of new processes and requires that you verify that all steps in the HRO safety system (Break-the-Chain Framework) have been successfully put in place before work on hazardous processes is begun.

- Once work begins, feedback at the *Tier 1 level* is obtained through ongoing and open communications between you and your employees. This feedback is focused on discovering potential hazards, identifying human error precursors, and determining the viability of defenses, and is intended to prevent errors before they can affect operations.

- *Tier 2* requires that you track and trend accumulated operations data. The intent here is to identify precursors to potential consequential events and allow corrective actions before a system accident occurs.

- If a system event or accident does occur, you can obtain *Tier 3* feedback by systematically

Chapter 6 | **133**

digging deeply into system operations to discover organizational factors that may have caused the unplanned occurrence.

- Finally, *Tier 4* enables you to apply information learned from significant events, accidents, and benchmarking practices external to your organization to your own operations.

Generating Decision-making Information: A Tiered Approach to Organizational Learning

Before you, as a manager, can make appropriate decisions about the effectiveness of your safety system, you must collect, evaluate, and interpret data. This is done through a system of feedback loops.

Feedback Loops: How Organizations Respond to Problems and Initiate Change

Feedback is an effective catalyst for organizational change. Organizations are complex systems that tend to be self stabilizing—they can replicate, repair, maintain, and reorganize themselves, and they tend to adjust to their environment. As a result, it is typically difficult for organizations to change. All dynamic organizational behavior is produced by a combination of reinforcing and balancing feedback loops:

- Reinforcing loops initiate change in one direction and then reinforce it with even more change in that direction. Such loops are often termed vicious or virtuous cycles.

- Balancing loops stabilize the system and resist change in one direction by producing change in the opposite direction to bring the system into equilibrium. If an organization resists change, a strong balancing dynamic is most likely present.

Feedback delays can add to system unpredictability and control difficulties because they make it difficult to understand the feedback, measure results, respond to a problem, and implement a solution. System managers may not even realize such delays exist.

Some systems are self regulating or adapting, that is, they use feedback loops that become ingrained. A feedback system can allow an organization to reactively reach a higher state of organization through learning, or feeding information into the process. This is an important notion for organizations desiring to refine their HRO systems. It may take many iterations to achieve the desired condition, but a controlled and measured approach using prediction, measurement, and continuous learning will keep the process moving forward.

Most complex organizations have many subsystems, which increase the challenges to change. Subsystems may have conflicting goals, or may even diverge from the overall system. Without the proper analysis and controls, feedback from a subsystem can be inaccurately conveyed or inaccurately interpreted.

To deal with this complexity, an HRO must use practices and approaches that allow it to process large quantities of information, learn quickly, act flexibly, and endure in spite of unpredictability in the environment. These practices are necessary to enable HROs to avoid system accidents and the associated catastrophic consequences. The tiered approach presented in the following sections explains how you can collect and transform raw data about your (and other) operations and transform this into information that will enable you to refine and improve your HRO system.

Tier 0: Program Start Up

Your first order of business as manager in a learning organization is to ensure that the HRO framework, essential for success, is fully integrated into all processes. This must occur before operations start up (Figure 6-1). Although Deming (1994) claimed that the most important aspect of the systems approach is the design of the system, a system must be implemented as designed to achieve the intended goals. Thus is it critical that you verify that all four HRO practices are in place before a new highly hazardous process is started. Essentially, this requires that you verify the presence of each component in the Break-the-Chain Framework before work begins (we call this Tier 0 because it should be accomplished before operational start up).

The level of rigor and formality used for start-up verification should be directly proportional to the complexity of the process and the consequence

Deviations from the norm can themselves be the norm.

(Dekker, 2006, p. 163)

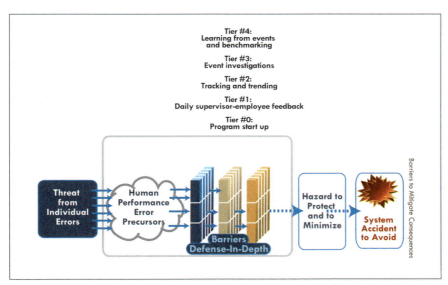

Figure 6-1. The Break-the-Chain Framework and the Tiered Approach to Organizational Learning

the organization is trying to prevent. For example, one would expect a more rigorous approach for the start up of a nuclear reactor, which in an accident scenario has the potential to affect the lives of thousands of people for many generations, than for a petroleum refinery.

Although laborious, start-up verification is actually the easiest part of the HRO feedback process from a reviewer's point of view. During start up, the organization bears the burden of proof to demonstrate that all processes, equipment, and training meet the established standards. It is not incumbent on the reviewing team to search out instances of noncompliance before start up; however, this start-up review is critical to high reliability operations. Organizational learning starts with process start-up verification. It provides the baseline against which everyday operations are judged. Weaknesses found at this tier should be viewed seriously; typically, things will only get worse as operations proceed and work becomes routine. Tracking and trending of start-up weaknesses indicates the seriousness of the organization's commitment to be an HRO and indicates whether the organization has the stamina to make all processes comply with the four HRO practices.

Tier 1: Daily Supervisor-Employee Feedback

As explained in Chapter 4, Break-the-Chain steps 3, 4, and 5 focus on recognizing and reducing human performance error precursors and on managing defenses to reduce operational threats to the existing hazard. This requires daily supervisor-employee interactions that provide immediate, real-time feedback on the successful management of human error precursors and flawed defenses (Figure 6-1).

Are you a line supervisor? If so, you should hold daily pre-work meetings with your staff. During these discussions, you should review the existing defensive barriers to determine if they are adequate to protect against a system accident: Are the barriers sufficient? Are they in place? Are they independently verified? Are they fully functional? How do you know these things? Additionally, you should discuss and evaluate any possible human performance error precursors that could affect your employees' capability to respond to unexpected events.

Keeping your employees aware of task demands such as time pressures and unexpected conditions will enable you and your staff to identify and address error-likely situations on the spot, thus reducing the likelihood of unexpected system occurrences. For example, one of your employees may admit to temporary limitations stemming from lack of sleep, sickness, or concerns at home; by sharing this information, the employee creates a healthy situation in which fellow employees can act as temporary back-up partners during critical steps in a process.

Other discussions you hold with your employees may help identify flawed or missing barriers that must be fixed before work commences. A prerequisite for this, however, is that your employees must know what barriers are supposed to be in place and understand how those various safety barriers are meant to function. Often, after many days of routine work with no events, employees start to relax and may begin to assume all barriers are in place without explicitly verifying their viability. To help your employees develop a mindset of chronic unease, you should require them to check all safety barriers on a daily basis.

Don't Hide Those Defenses!

Safety barriers that employees don't know about or understand are often violated and seldom effective. As a manager, take care that you:

- Don't hide barriers from your employees.

- Continually prompt employees to verify the existence and the effectiveness of barriers.

Your employees need to understand which barriers are meant to defend against which hazards. After all, they have the most to lose if an ineffective or missing barrier leads to systemic failure.

> *"The problem with complex, dynamic worlds is that safety is not constant. Past success while departing from the routine is not a guarantee for future safety. In other words, a safe outcome today is not a guarantee of a safe outcome tomorrow, even if behavior is the same."*
>
> *(Dekker, 2006, p. 164)*

Because work is dynamic, the feedback process between you and your employees must continue as the work shift progresses. If any barriers are found missing, or breached, or if additional signs of human error precursors surface, you must suspend work and make sure the situation is immediately remedied. Barriers to protect against the system accident are not put in place to be challenged everyday because of sloppy work, they are put in place to protect the plant from the employee when the employee has a bad day. As such, signs of challenged barriers should be taken as a warning sign of poor operations. The key to this process is to maintain open two-way communications between yourself and your employees.

Two primary tools that you can use to help identify human performance error precursors and ensure hazards are adequately defended are the TWIN Analysis Matrix and the Barrier Analysis Matrix. These tools are also employed during CFA investigations to help compile and organize data about the failure modes of the system event being studied.[9]

As used here, the TWIN Analysis Matrix is a proactive tool in Step 3 of the Break-the-Chain Framework (Chapter 4). It helps to identify and categorize human error precursors before and during work to determine which situations or factors stretch the employee beyond his ability to adapt. For example, are you, as an employee responsible for a particular job, overwhelmed by the demands of the task, the work environment, your own limited individual capabilities, or other human conditions? The TWIN Matrix, shown in Figure 4-6, is used to the tabulate results of such an analysis by category. This provides a summary of where corrective intervention should

Chapter 6 | **139**

be focused to preclude error-likely situations for a given individual or operation.

As shown in Figure 6-2, the Barrier Analysis Matrix is a five-column table that managers and employees can use to describe and track the performance of the various defensive barriers. Each barrier is analyzed to determine the target (hazard) it protects, the threat it protects against (individual error), and the effectiveness of the barrier against the intended threat. The significance of any weakness exhibited by the barrier is then considered in terms of its possible contribution to a system event or accident. For example, if the hazard is the presence of explosive materials, a defensive barrier could be to ensure that all flame initiators, such as cigarette lighters, are prohibited from the area. Thus, all employees entering this area must deposit cigarette lighters at the entrance. To determine the effectiveness of the barrier, you might perform a quick check of all employees' pockets before

> A system is a network of interdependent components working together to accomplish a specific aim. The greater the interdependence between components, the greater the need for communication and cooperation among these components and the greater the need for overall management.
>
> *(Deming, 1994)*

Barrier	Hazard Protected	Threat	Effectiveness of Barrier	Significance
①	②	③	④	⑤

STEPS TO POPULATE:

1. List the barrier in Column 1.
2. List the hazard the barrier is supposed to protect in Column 2.
3. List the threat in Column 3 (note these may be all the same for a single event).
4. Describe how effective barrier was in protecting target from threat in Column 4.
5. Describe the significance of the failed barrier to this event in Column 5.

Figure 6-2. Barrier Analysis Matrix (Corcoran, 2007)

> *People feel stress when they perceive a mismatch between problem demands and coping resources. One consequence of stress is tunneling—the tendency to see an increasingly narrow portion of one's operating environment. Another consequence is regression—the tendency to revert to earlier learned routines even if not entirely appropriate to the current situation.*
>
> *(Dekker, 2006, p. 142)*

any high explosives work is started. A flawed barrier—that is, the failure of employees to leave lighters or other flame sources at the door to the area—could contribute significantly to the likelihood of a high-explosives detonation.

The Tier 1 feedback loop is indirectly discussed in Break-the-Chain Step 6 (Chapter 4), which focuses on evaluating and closing the gap between the work-as-imagined by management and work-as-done by the employee. Key to this type of feedback is communication. Employees at every level of an HRO should seek to continuously communicate opportunities for improvement related to their own performance, equipment performance, the work environment, and organizational processes. This communication is particularly important at the manager/first-line supervisor/employee interface because it is here, where employees touch the plant, that active errors occur and can be prevented. As a manager, you can promote continuous improvement in the organization's culture through responsiveness to your employees' operational and safety concerns. Open communication channels will help you be aware of problems that exist in your work area and provide you with ideas about how to correct them. Trust is generated by your effort to actively address your employees' concerns.

Tier 2: Tracking and Trending

In addition to daily feedback obtained from your employees, as a manager you must ensure that routine monitoring of the HRO framework is performed. This allows your organization to collect, track, trend, and understand the performance data in terms of the measures of effectiveness (discussed in Chapter 7) for each of the HRO practices.

The usefulness of routine performance data hinges on how well they can be used to identify common operational trends or deficiencies in the safety system that could eventually degrade its ability to protect against system accidents. In essence, the collected and analyzed data should be a means of monitoring the health of the HRO organizational system. Too often, however, monitoring data collected by high-hazard operations focuses on outcome measures that may not be useful for this purpose. As noted by James Reason (1997, p. 107), a professor of psychology at Manchester University in England:

"Most organizations involved in hazardous operations rely heavily upon outcome measures, or specifically, upon negative outcome measures that record the occurrence of adverse events such as fatalities and lost time injuries.

Outcome data provide an unreliable indication of a system's intrinsic safety. Only if the managers of a system had complete control over all possible accident-producing factors could negative outcome data provide a valid index of its intrinsic safety. Natural hazards can be defended against, unsafe acts can be moderated to some degree, but neither can be eliminated altogether. Latent conditions, or pathogens, will always be present. The likelihood of their adverse conjunction is always greater than zero.

Outcome data can only reveal the negative face of safety. Such measures record moments of vulnerability; they cannot discriminate the more enduring ingredients of resistance. These need to be assessed directly using process measures—indices that gauge the general safety health of the system as a whole by sampling various vital signs on a regular basis" (Reason, 1997).

This quote from Reason illustrates why the tracking of individual safety statistics alone does

Gap Between Work-as-imagined And Work-as-done

"The problem is not that different images of work exist. Problems arise when the organization is not sufficiently aware of the gap between these images. Having a gap is not an indication of a dysfunctional organization. But not knowing about it, and not learning why it exists, is."

(Dekker, 2006, p. 168)

Counting Errors

Counting errors and stuffing them away in a measurement instrument (and handing the results to management in the form of a bar chart) removes the context. It is gone, no longer there.

- Without context, you cannot reconstruct local rationality.

- Without local rationality, you cannot understand human error.

- So counting error is contrary to understanding error.

(Dekker, 2006, p. 68)

not indicate the success of an HRO in preventing a catastrophic event. Such statistics may indicate moments of vulnerability of the organizational system; if the individual safety statistics (total recordable or lost-time accidents) are poor, this likely indicates the HRO is having problems. However, good safety statistics say nothing about how capable the HRO is with respect to avoiding a system accident (refer to the Columbia accident). To provide positive indicators, measures of effectiveness must be established using specific lines of inquiry along with specific thresholds or measures of success. These lines of inquiry and corresponding measures of effectiveness must be used sparingly, as the cost to acquire such data is high and wearing on the participants (none of us want to be accused of crying wolf or of acting like Chicken Little). In Chapter 7, we present specific measures of effectiveness for each HRO practice.

The following is an example of how you might develop a line of inquiry and a measure of effectiveness for ensuring that the safety system provides safety (one of the actions required under HRO Practice 1). This particular positive measure of effectiveness focuses on ensuring sufficient technical expertise as determined by the needs of your process. You would want to make sure that existing managers, as they change positions due to rotations, are replaced with managers who have the appropriate technical education and/or experience to understand how to sustain the culture of reliability (i.e., optimize the product output while maintaining the safety envelope). This measure could be expressed quantitatively as a percentage of the total number of newly-assigned managers. For example, if your organization deals with nuclear hazards, your process may require that a significant percent of the managers have nuclear engineering degrees with the appropriate level of experience. A decrease in this percentage of technically-qualified managers over time or a decrease below your established threshold (e.g., dropping below 85 percent), without a corresponding change in your processes, could indicate a reduction in your ability to avoid a consequential event. This indicator would be a sort of early warning flag, apparent well in advance of any detrimental effects on the organization.

Tier 3: Event Investigations

Tier 3 involves using the Causal Factors Analysis process to systematically investigate and understand the role of human performance and organizational weaknesses in system events. An accident is not a prerequisite for this tier; discrete, low- or no-consequence events (we call them *information-rich events*) can provide a wealth of information about systemic problems if you are willing to spend the time to discover the underlying reasons why the event occurred (the why behind the what). This is shown graphically in Figure 6-3 (on the following page) which indicates how an investigation works backward from the event to determine its causes. Essentially, then, the CFA process works in reverse to the factors that led up to the event (Figure 4-4). By taking this top-down approach to separate what happened from why it happened, the CFA investigation systematically identifies the flawed defenses, the active failures, the human performance error precursors, and, eventually, the latent conditions that set up the event.

Event investigations exist for two main reasons. First, the investigation aims to stop recurrence of the event or similar events that could lead to

---

What Qualifies As An Information-rich Event?

Any system that:

(1) discloses a significant gap between work-as-imagined and work-as-done;

(2) is a new type of event (or the result of a new type of error) not afforded protection by the system; or

(3) is an event that could have resulted in significant consequences.

This determination is very intuitive. Trust your gut.

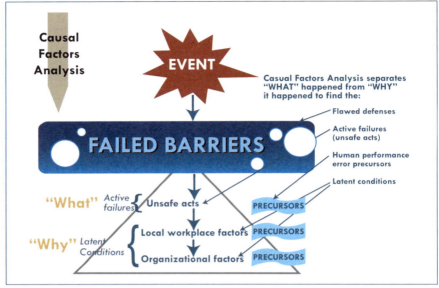

Figure 6-3. Causal Factors Analysis to Determine Organizational Weaknesses (Reason, 1997)

significant consequences the next time around. Second, it helps the organization learn about itself as an HRO.

The CFA process essentially requires the investigators to work through the Break-the-Chain Framework in reverse, looking for failures that caused or contributed to the chain of events that preceded the occurrence. The idea is this: if the steps in the Break-the-Chain Framework could have prevented the system event, then, once an event occurs, the logical way to find out where the system broke down is to work through the steps of the Break-the-Chain Framework in reverse. Figure 6-4 notes how the CFA investigation team examines the framework systematically, identifying any weaknesses or deficiencies along the way; the white numbers (inside blue circles) in this figure indicate the sequence used to conduct the investigation:

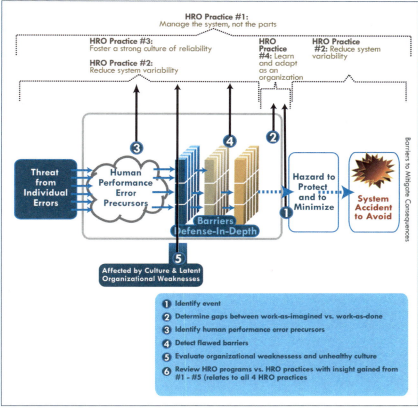

Figure 6-4. Output of Causal Factors Analysis to Evaluate HRO Practices

1. The event facts surrounding the event and the initiating actions are identified using the timeline tools described in *Causal Factors Analysis: An Approach to Organizational Learning* (Hartley et al., 2008).

2. Comparative timelines are used to identify gaps between work-as-imagined and work-as-done. These gaps provide insight as to the effectiveness of programs that support HRO Practice 4.

3. Human performance error precursors are identified using a comparative timeline

Accident Models And Their Constraints

- In a sequence-of-events model, the choice of events considered causal to one another are subjective and always incomplete. Often, the human link is painted as the weakest link.

- Epidemiological models can allow the search for latent pathogens to escalate out of control; in an extreme application of this model nearly everything inside an organization could be construed as a possible latent failure. Thus, although the model is useful in discovering latent failures after a mishap occurs, it is more difficult to make meaningful predictions with it.

- Systemic models explain accidents in terms of inadequate control over interactions between components and processes, but as Dekker says, "because our systems are growing increasingly complex, such interactions are difficult to model" and "inadequate control over them is not easy to define."

(Dekker, 2006, p. 81)

and the TWIN Analysis Matrix. These precursors provide feedback as to the effectiveness of programs used to support HRO Practice 3 by indicating mismatches between an employee's ability and the stresses of the work environment. Large gaps indicate the employee is not prepared to effectively execute or make decisions to meet management expectations.

4. Flawed defenses are detected through a Barrier Analysis; these indicate the effectiveness of programs developed to support HRO Practice 2. Both managers and employees need to be aware of and understand the safety barriers. As the responsible manager, you should provide the information you have about barriers that were penetrated and/or missing to the CFA investigation team; this will provide insight as to areas that should be improved immediately to protect the workforce.

5. Latent organizational weaknesses and cultural factors that set up the situation leading to this event are reviewed against the programs that support HRO Practice 1 to evaluate which programs are working. This is a challenging comparison because of the abstract nature of HRO Practice 1. To understand the weaknesses in the organization and HRO framework, all information must be rolled up and the individual causal factors must be extrapolated to the organizational level. Information that is available at the conclusion of the CFA investigation to help with this extrapolation includes:

    - Knowledge of the organization-specific HRO practices and programs.

Chapter 6   147

- A list of the causal factors.

- A list of those factors that did not cause the event but require fixing, ECAQ and their associated corrective actions, and LTBL.

- Cultural insight.

- An understanding of the significance of the human performance error precursors.

- An evaluation of the significance of the flawed defenses and remaining barriers.

- An evaluation of how long the problem has gone undetected and uncorrected in the organization.

- An understanding of the size of the gaps between work-as-imagined and work-as-done.

The entire CFA process includes five discrete steps as shown in the CFA flowchart in Figure 6-5:

- Event recognition

- Investigation

- Analysis

- Corrective actions

- Learning

Step-by-step instructions on the process as well as suggested tools and examples to carry out the steps are presented in the companion volume to this guide, *Causal Factors Analysis: An Approach to Organizational Learning* (Hartley et al. 2008).

Tier 4: Learning from External Events and Benchmarking

The last tier in this approach involves exploiting the wealth of information available from external system accident investigations (i.e., those

---

Don't Wait For An Accident!
Nonconsequential, information-rich events can provide as much insight into organizational weaknesses as accidents—perhaps even more, considering that the involved employees are still around to interview.

Cause
Cause is not something you find but something you construct. How you construct it and what evidence you use depends on:

- Where you look

- What you look for

- To whom you talk

- What you have seen before

- More than likely, who your boss is

(Dekker, 2006, p. 76)

that occur in other organizations) and from benchmarking best HRO practices developed by other organizations or at the industry level.

Unfortunately, the list of system accident case studies is not small. It includes such examples as the industrial disaster in Bhopal, India; the explosions of the space shuttles Challenger and Columbia; the nuclear disaster at Chernobyl, Ukraine; and many others.

To enable those in your organization to learn from these major accidents, we recommend evaluating select accident investigations using the six pitfalls of the Break-the-Chain Framework noted in Chapter 4 as a guide. These pitfalls are:

- Losing focus and forgetting about the consequences.
- Failing to recognize and minimize the hazard.
- Losing sight of the threat posed by human error.

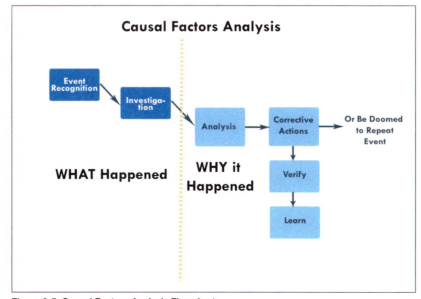

Figure 6-5. Causal Factors Analysis Flowchart

- Failing to recognize and minimize human performance error precursors.

- Failing to manage defenses.

- Failing to identify and minimize the gap between work-as-imagined and work-as-done.

A key component in researching external accidents is to determine what type of system the organization had in place before the accident. Often, the point is not that the organization was unsafe–it may have had some of the best safety practices in place at the time. More likely, the organization became complacent as a result of the long intervals of time during which there were no significant events. How to fight complacency, a normal human tendency when things are going well, is the greatest challenge of any HRO. Learning from other organization's accidents is a way of maintaining or refreshing the chronic unease of your organization in its fight against complacency.

Benchmarking best practices is another powerful tool that should be considered in strategic planning for HRO improvement. Best practices are strategies and techniques employed by top performers in a given industry. Since top performers are not generally the best in class in every area related to their industry, it is important to target areas in your organization that you know are in need of improvement, then select an organization in your industry whose performance in these areas is exemplary as the model or benchmark. Using detailed gap analyses, you can implement action plans that compare your facility practices, on an ongoing basis, with those of best-in-class organizations. The implementation of changes resulting from benchmarking

Commonalities Among Major System Accidents*:

- Divided responsibilities for operations

- Mindset that success is routine

- Belief that rule compliance is sufficient

- Team player emphasis limits dissent

- Experience from other fields neglected

- Lessons learned neglected

- Safety issues subordinate to other goals

- Emergency drills and procedures neglected

- Known hazardous design features allowed

- Known risk management methods unused

- Ambiguous jurisdictions for safety integration

(Zebroski, 2003)

* Bhopal chemical release, Challenger shuttle booster failure, Chernobyl reactor runaway and explosion, Houston chemical complex explosions, Piper Alpha platform fire and explosions, rocket fuel organization fire and explosions, Three Mile Island-2 meltdown.

should include an overall strategy to make your employees aware of the need, urgency, methodology, and responsibilities for changing a facility process to match that of a benchmarked organization. Adopting a new process should be carried out using specific objectives that are tied to eliminating identified weaknesses in the identified process.

Integrate and Interpret Feedback to Enable Better Decision Making

Once feedback data has been generated using a tiered approach, you, as a manager, need to help your organization:

- Determine the level of significance this feedback has to the organization.

- Extrapolate singular event data to the organizational level.

- Compare results between system events to identify cycles.

- Use this information to evaluate and make decisions about the effectiveness of the four HRO practices in your organization.

Evaluate Organizational Significance

Evaluating how the individual data points collected from the five tiers function as a part of the bigger picture contributes to your understanding of why system accidents and events occur (Figure 6-1). This allows you, as a manager, to make fact-based predictions and corrections that are informed by knowledge of the interdependence of the system, as described by Deming's principle of the knowledge of variation (1994). The level of significance is based on several factors:

- Size of the gap between work-as-imagined and work-as-done

- Likelihood that the event is a precursor to other, perhaps more significant, events
- Number of flawed or missing defenses and the robustness of remaining barriers
- Pervasiveness of the problem in time or space
- Impact of the event on the credibility of the organization, as viewed by the customer

For example, the level of significance for feedback obtained at the Tier 3 level (event investigations) indicates how rich (in information) a given event was to the HRO and how much time and effort should be afforded to remedying the problems indicated by the event.

Extrapolate Singular Event Data to the Organizational Level

As noted in Chapter 5, the culture of a group is a pattern of shared, basic assumptions that was learned by the group as it solved problems of external adaptation and internal integration (Schein 1992). Because the behavior of employee reflects the organizational culture, it is possible to extrapolate singular events to the organizational level by comparing the event characteristics to common organizational weaknesses. These latent organizational weaknesses—that is, hidden deficiencies in processes (such as strategy, policies, work control, training, and resource allocation) or values (shared beliefs, attitudes, norms, and assumptions)—create workplace conditions that can provoke active human error and degrade the integrity of the system defenses. Such weaknesses are identified by comparing causal factors to the common organizational weaknesses shown in Table 6-1, found on page 154.

Pondering the possible existence of these latent organizational weaknesses within your

---

Nobody Has The Time To Participate In Benchmarking Studies Any More

- The number one reason, surprisingly, wasn't time (that finished at number four)—it was a lack of resources. Without enough people (and the right people) to participate in benchmarking activities, and certainly without a sufficient budget, companies' efforts to benchmark are doomed before they even get started.

- The number two reason was that internal measures and processes are difficult to define—if you don't know what you want to measure, then how can you ever discern if what you're doing is up to industry standards?

- The third most prevalent deterrent to benchmarking is the difficulty in identifying proper benchmarking partners.

(Grenoble, 2005)

Story Of The Boiling Frog

"It is said that if a frog is placed in boiling water, it will jump out, but if is placed in cold water that is slowly heated, it will never jump out and will end up being boiled alive.

The story is told in a figurative context, with the upshot being that people should make themselves aware of gradual change lest they suffer a catastrophic loss."

(Wikipedia, 2008)

"A safety culture is a culture that allows the boss to hear bad news."

(Dekker, 2006, p. 171)

---

organization should motivate you to review your current management practices and processes (and those of your organization) to look for potential set-up factors that could result in a consequential accident. To ensure your review is comprehensive, the latent organizational weaknesses listed in Table 6-1 are cross-referenced to the various elements of the McKinsey 7S approach (Peters and Waterman, 1982) introduced in Chapter 3. In this way, if you discover an organizational weakness associated with the implementing strategies used during the transition process you can be assured that your organization either made an incomplete gap analysis, developed inappropriate strategies, or incompletely executed the strategies to close the identified gaps between its pre-HRO state and the desired HRO end state. This is good feedback for you as a manager of a learning organization.

Compare Results Between System Events to Discover Cycles

Employees and managers come and go. Organizations learn and forget. Because of the cyclical nature of organizational learning, it is important to review and integrate information from each of the five feedback tiers over time and across the entire organization. This may provide an indication of a negative trend or dangerous cycle that would not otherwise be detected. The identification of such trends could provide you with the warning needed to avoid a system accident.

Evaluate the Effectiveness of the HRO Practices

The last step in converting feedback data to decision-making information is to evaluate the ability of your management system to support and sustain HRO practices. This involves comparing all the information described above against the HRO programs to evaluate their effectiveness in instituting the four HRO practices. For example, an evaluation of human performance error precursors and flawed defenses can be used to gauge the effectiveness of HRO Practice 2 and the programs you instituted to carry it out. An evaluation of the culture of reliability and latent organizational weaknesses can be used to gauge the effectiveness of HRO Practice 3 and its associated programs. The gap between work-as-imagined and work-as-done can be used to evaluate HRO Practice 4. Finally, the integration and interpretation of all the feedback information can be used to evaluate HRO Practice 1. Any weaknesses or lack of stellar performance in the respective programs may indicate a need to refine the system to improve safety.

Refine the HRO System: Apply a Systems Approach to Reduce Variability

We talked in Chapter 4 about modifying individual processes within the HRO system; in this section, we address how to modify the system as a whole. The last step in instituting HRO Practice 4 is to refine the HRO system based on feedback about your organization's culture of reliability and latent organizational weaknesses. This reflects Deming's (1994) emphasis on understanding and reducing variability in the system and using feedback as the basis for learning.

Insight into your organization's culture of reliability represents a roll-up of the individual factors observed during an event investigation; in essence, it is a snapshot that indicates how pervasive the identified conditions are across the organization. A culture whose unwritten rules are at odds with those needed to ensure safety and reliability can negatively impact operations.

Table 6-1. Common Organizational Weaknesses*

Category	McKinsey 7S Approach**	Weakness
Training	Skills	• Lack of effective training • No task qualification requirement when the task is skill-based • Focus on lower level of cognitive knowledge • Failure to have management involved in training • Training not consistent with organization equipment, procedures, or process
Communication	Systems	• Failure to reinforce use of the phonetic alphabet • Failure to reinforce use of 3-way communications • Failure to use specific unit ID numbers in procedures • Unclear priorities or expectations • Unclear roles and responsibilities
Planning and Scheduling	Systems	• Not anticipating failures and providing contingencies • Not considering multiple components out of service • Not providing required materials or procedures • Over scheduling resources • Tunnel vision/failure to consider incorrect operation or damage to adjacent equipment • Specific type of work not performed • Specific type of issue not addressed • Inadequate resources assigned
Design or Process Change	Strategy	• Inadequate involvement of users in design change implementation • Inadequate training • Inadequate contingencies

continued

Chapter 6 | 155

Table 6-1. Common Organizational Weaknesses*

Category	McKinsey 7S Approach**	Weakness
Values, Priorities, Policies	Shared Values	• Management polices discourage line input • Too high priority placed on schedules • Willingness to accept degraded conditions or performance • Management failure to recognize the need for or importance of related program
Procedure Development or Use	Systems	• Human factors not considered in procedure development and implementation • Failure to perform procedure verification or validation • Failure to reference procedure during task performance • Assumptions made in lieu of procedure guidance • Omission of necessary functions in procedures
Supervisory Involvement	Style/Staff	• Failure to perform management observations and coaching • Not correcting poor performance or reinforcing good performance • Unassigned or fragmented responsibility and accountability • Inadequate program oversight
Organizational Interfaces	Structure	• Unclear interfaces for defining work priorities • Lack of clear lines of communications between organizations • Conflicting goals or requirements between programs • Lack of self assessment monitoring • Lack of measurement tools for monitoring program performance • Lack of interface between programs
Work Practices	Systems	• Failure to reinforce use of established error prevention tools and techniques (human performance tools)

*Used with permission, TXU, 2005
**Peters and Waterman, 1982

For example, as shown in Figure 6-6, critical safety requirements could be ignored when the culture of reliability is not in alignment with the requirements for high reliability operations, thus increasing safety risks. Insight into the culture helps us understand how unwritten organizational rules may preclude adherence to established safety requirements and how corrective actions or the application of lessons to be learned (LTBL) can help align the culture with the stated organizational goals and requirements.

As an HRO manager, you have deployed a system approach to prevent a system accident. Accordingly, when things don't go according to plan, you need to look at the underlying system, not just the last person in the chain of events.[10] Anderson and Johnson (1997) provide a useful approach to problem solving that is based on systems thinking. This approach encourages organizations to examine the larger picture, structure, and relationships to explain an employee's behavior. It emphasizes that each component and person in the organization contributes to problems in the system. Such problems can be solved through an approach that includes the following steps:

- Formulate the problem.

- Identify the variables.

- Prioritize the variables (plan the order of attack).

- Define each variable precisely.

- Create a hypothesis to explain the problematic behavior.

- Track and revise reasoning.

- Test possible solutions.

- Reformulate the problem based on the new understanding gained.

A systems approach to problem solving enables you, as a manager, to recognize general patterns of behavior and the structures that produce them, which helps you to identify underlying problems. Chronic, unresolved problems are more often the result of systemic breakdowns, not individual mistakes; thus, if the goal is to successfully solve a problem, managers must understand the structure that is causing the problem. You should be wary of a symptomatic fix disguised as a long-term, high-leverage intervention. Also, because learning

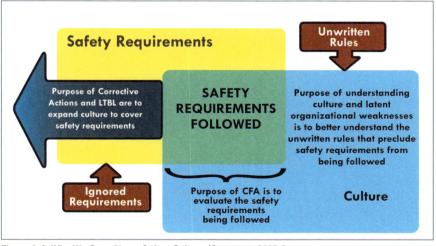

Figure 6-6. Why We Care About Safety Culture (Corcoran, 2007d)

is an iterative process, once you formulate a solution, you must follow up with an evaluation of results and outcomes from a systemic perspective.

To help align results of organizational programs with your organization's stated goals and requirements, we recommend deploying Six Sigma and Lean techniques to continually optimize the system. The continued refinement of the HRO system will keep it viable and reduce the opportunity for complacency. In a fixed resource environment, the more optimized the processes, the more time is available to focus on safety.

Chapter 7

Chapter 7

Evaluating Your Organization's Culture of Reliability: Determine the Effectiveness of the HRO Practices

This chapter answers the following questions:

- How do I characterize my organization's culture of reliability?

- How can I use this characterization to evaluate my organization's culture of reliability?

- What does the health of my organization's culture of reliability tell me about the effectiveness of my HRO?

- If I discover indications of an unhealthy culture, how can I go about improving it?

Throughout this guide we have discussed the four HRO practices that an organization should implement to become an HRO and to sustain high reliability operations. We have held off in providing specific measures to evaluate the effectiveness of each practice because we believe that these practices, like the elements of Deming's Theory of Knowledge (1994), are not separate elements in the HRO system, but represent interrelated and nested actions that vary in sequence or emphasis depending on the dynamics of the organization and the situations faced daily. Thus, it is nearly impossible to evaluate the individual components or practices of your organization's HRO system.

We believe the effectiveness of your HRO system hinges on how well your organization's culture of reliability supports the four HRO practices. Hence, to evaluate your organization's performance as an HRO, you must observe your organization's culture of reliability, as reflected in the behaviors, espoused values, and intrinsic beliefs of its employees. Does this culture reflect those behaviors, values, and underlying assumptions that you, as a manager, want your organization to aspire to as an HRO?

To help you in this evaluation, we first describe how you can characterize your culture of reliability. That is what are the signs you should look for to help you describe this important feature of your organization? Next, we provide lines of inquiry and suggested measures of effectiveness to use the characterization you have made as an evaluation tool, to determine how your organization's culture of reliability relates to the four HRO practices. By providing you with specific types of probing questions, our intent is to enable you to determine how well your organization is performing each HRO practice and whether these practices are resulting in the desired outcomes. Finally, we present some suggestions about what you can do if you discover your organization has an unhealthy culture.

Characterize Your Organization's Culture of Reliability

Knowing how to characterize your organization's culture of reliability—that is, how to recognize and describe those features that pertain to high reliability operations—is a daunting task. The exact categories or attributes you choose to highlight are not as important as your struggle to better recognize and understand what the signs of a culture of reliability are within the context of your operations and what they indicate about your organization's ability to implement and sustain the four HRO practices.

William Corcoran (2007a) has parsed this characterization process into simple, recognizable indicators that an astute observer would notice when walking around the worksite. Your organization's culture, according to William Corcoran, can be characterized using four primary indicators, as shown in Figure 7-1 and described in more detail in the following sections:

- *Shared mental content*
- *Norms*
- *Institution*
- *Physical items*

Shared Mental Content

Shared mental content consists of such intangible things such as beliefs, values, cognitive models, unwritten rules, attitudes, prejudices, mental short cuts, rules-of-thumb, skills, accepted fallacies, tribal knowledge, paradigms, heuristics, and any other identifiable mental concepts or tools that are generally shared among members of the group. For example, some faith communities share a belief in "the Golden Rule." This belief is shared mental content.

Another example of shared mental content is the adage, once a prevalent attitude among retailers and service companies, that "The customer is always right." (When put into practice, this shared mental attitude would be a norm. If it were written down in an employee-training course, it would also become a physical item.) The industrial operations mantra of Stop-Think-Act-Review is another example of what we hope is a prevalent

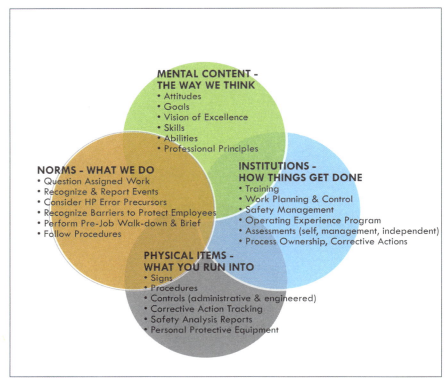

Figure 7-1. Characterization of Safety Culture (Corcoran, 2007a)

shared mental approach to conducting high-hazard operations.

The synchronization of the shared mental content of a group with the artifacts or behaviors observed in the individual members is a good indicator of a culture of reliability (i.e., a healthy safety culture) and a characteristic worth noting.

Norms

A norm is a behavior that typically occurs in a specified situation. Norms include language, traditions, rituals, customs, and similar behaviors. For example, saying grace before a meal is a norm in some families.

Norms can be observed and recorded, whereas mental content cannot be observed directly. There is not always a one-to-one mapping of shared mental content and observable norms.

It may well be that a common language is a foundational norm for a culture, since language is a key medium for transmitting mental content, norms, institutional processes, and written physical items. Language includes vocabulary, formality, uniformity, lingo, jargon, and the like. The use of a particular language indicates both shared mental content and an observable norm. When the language is written, it is revealed as a physical item. For example:

- Communications that occur in an aircraft's flight deck and between the aircraft and flight controllers are characterized by the use of the International Phonetic Alphabet (Alpha, Bravo, Charlie…). This is an observable norm among pilots. This norm is not observed consistently among airline employees who are not pilots, not even in situations where error rates could be reduced by the use of this language.

- In certain private schools, the students stand up when a faculty member enters the classroom. This norm is not observed in public schools.

- In Quaker meetings, applause, although rarely rendered, is indicated when members of the group hold up their hands and shake and rotate them. This norm produces no sound and seems consistent with the Quakers' reverence for silence.

- In some cultures, men and women eat in different rooms; however, in contemporary

American culture, men and women eat together. Both behaviors are observable norms.

Some norms are hierarchical or rank-based. In other words, they may apply to certain levels of the organization, but not to others. For example, executives in an organization may eat in a special dining room. Some norms are classification-based; for example, salaried professionals do not punch a time clock.

Institutions

Institutions are the formal structures and processes by which an organization carries out its activities across the entire organization in a consistent fashion. For example, during the early nineteenth century, the Plains Indians of the American West harvested North American bison using an institution called the hunting party. Likewise, medieval Christianity provided religious services to its members by the institution called the priesthood and the U.S. Government collects most of its taxes through an institution called the Internal Revenue Service. In New England, many communities still make important decisions by means of an institution called the Town Meeting, even though this term has been borrowed for less formal purposes.

In organizations characterized by high-hazard operations, there are hundreds of institutions that are recognized as programs. Each of these is a separate institution. For example, some high-hazard industries have corrective action programs for formally processing problems and improvement opportunities. These programs are institutions that are part of the organizational culture. Other institutions may include configuration management, drawing update, labeling, industrial hygiene, hearing protection, employee concerns, and employee assistance.

In summary, the following can be identified as institutions:

- Named subgroups (the Town Council, the Capital Project Review Committee)

- Named processes (a land use review hearing, a wedding)

- Named gatherings (a cocktail party, a plan-of-the-day meeting)

- Named programs (the In-Service Inspection Program, the Quality Assurance Program)

- Named positions (the Town Manager, Chief Engineer, Certified Safety Professional, or Causal Factors Analysis Team Leader)

Characteristic Physical Items

Characteristic physical items are those tangible entities that are characteristic of a culture. These items may have a variety of origins and purposes, but all are typical of the culture in which they are found. For example, most of the known American Indian tribes produced stone arrowheads in the past. Native Mesoamerican groups often had sacrifice altars; however, native North Americans did not.

An important subset of physical items includes signs, symbols, totems, and similar meaningful objects. For example, Protestants display a bare cross, whereas Roman Catholics display a crucifix. Submarine sailors wear dolphins, but aviators wear wings. In the modern U.S. culture, we encounter tattoos, facial jewelry, cellular telephones, and iPods—some of which are more or less prevalent, depending on the age group represented.

Physical items affect behaviors and thereby affect norms. For example, pre-work briefs conducted in hot, noisy, dusty rooms are likely to be short and probably incomplete. To improve the effectiveness of these briefs, you—the manager—should change the physical situation. Speed bumps and rumble strips are other physical items that affect norms. By requiring drivers to slow down, these features encourage norms consistent with safe driving.

In some high-hazard industries, personnel wear badge-sized identification cards. These are characteristic physical items, but the wearing of them would be a norm. Other examples of physical items in a high-hazard industry include signage (i.e., hazardous warning signs, confined space signs, safety awareness signs, etc.), the existence and use of written procedures, and various types of engineering and administrative controls to protect the hazard from the employee (e.g., safety analysis reports and personal protective equipment).

Evaluate Your Organization's Culture of Reliability

Armed with Corcoran's indicators (2007a) for characterizing safety culture, we can now turn our attention to how you can use these indicators/characteristics to determine if there are issues with your organization's culture of reliability that need to be addressed. This is a complicated subject which we have attempted to simplify by proceeding in steps. First, we describe how to evaluate a culture of reliability. Next, we use previously presented information to develop specific lines of inquiry that help focus discussions. Finally, we introduce the need for metrics to help you measure the relative health of your organization's culture of reliability.

Evaluating Your Culture of Reliability

A culture of reliability has two major requirements (Figure 7-2):

- The underlying assumptions of the managers are aligned with their espoused values.

- The espoused values of the managers are aligned with the behaviors and artifacts exhibited by its members.

This emphasizes why it is crucial for the managers of an HRO to walk the talk. Your espoused values should not represent only those items you talk about continuously, your espoused values should be visible in the actions you take every day. It is easy to talk the company line about safety; it is totally different and much harder to live this same company line. But beware! Any perceived or actual misalignments between the values you voice and those you act on will be noted by your employees and will quickly erode their trust in the

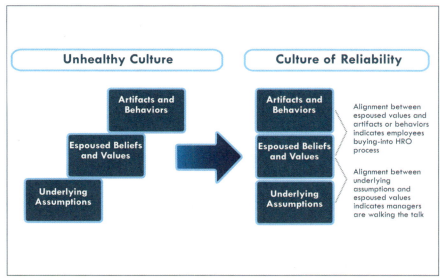

Figure 7-2. Culture of Reliability

HRO system your organization is trying so hard to implement (and, perhaps, also their trust in you as a manager).

Figure 7-2 illustrates how alignment or misalignment of underlying assumptions, espoused values and observable behaviors is used to indicate the health of a culture of reliability. It is crucial for the success of an HRO that observable indicators (e.g., norms, institutions, and physical items) within the organization align with the espoused beliefs and values of the organization. For an HRO, these espoused values are the four HRO practices as adapted and implemented by the organization. This makes the evaluation of safety culture, if done systematically and with forethought, a powerful feedback tool about the effectiveness of the HRO practices put in place to avoid the consequential system accident.

The evaluation of your organization's culture is an integral view; it examines both the behavior of the entire organization and indirect indicators of behavior that result from some of the HRO programs that have been instituted. To complete this evaluation, you must be armed with a fundamental understanding of the attributes that characterize a culture of reliability; this information will help you interpret what you observe and develop functional lines of inquiry that are aligned with the four HRO practices.

Use Lines of Inquiry to Highlight Areas for Improvement

Table 7-1 presents lines of inquiry and suggested metrics to help you evaluate whether your organization's artifacts and behaviors adequately align with the four HRO practices (which should represent the espoused beliefs and values of management within an HRO). The lines of inquiry originated from existing research by William Corcoran (2007a) and the Nuclear Regulatory Commission (2006), but have been modified and expanded based on the concepts presented in this guide. The metrics, which are presented only as guidelines, were developed through our own experience as managers of high-hazard operations and are discussed in the following section.

The lines of inquiry are intended to be used as a means of helping you evaluate, through systematic observations of the behaviors of your organization, the effectiveness of the HRO practices you have adopted and implemented to avoid the system accident. There are no right or wrong answers; the intent of this evaluation is to help you consider your organization's culture of reliability objectively. A few examples of questions you may ask include:

- Which aspects of our HRO program does the management team really buy into as evidenced by their actions, not just their words?

- What aspects of the HRO program do our employees buy into?

- What aspects of our organization's current culture provide us with the stamina needed to be successful as an HRO?

- What aspects of our current culture inhibit the effective implementation of the desired HRO practices?

Although the list of lines of inquiry may seem long, keep in mind that you don't need to apply all of them to every review. Their main purpose is to encourage you to think carefully about and question various aspects of your organization's current safety behaviors and beliefs. Some lines of inquiry may not be applicable to your operation; feel free to use whatever combination works best for you. The lines of inquiry presented in Table 7-1 are the foundation for the evaluation of culture of reliability as discussed in this guide and its companion volume, *Causal Factors Analysis: An Approach for Organizational Learning* (Hartley et al., 2008).

Use Meaningful Metrics to Evaluate Performance

Metrics are key to successful management; you can't manage what you can't measure (Deming, 1994). Once you begin to appreciate what the results of your operational practices of an HRO will look like, you can begin to develop specific measures to determine the relative effectiveness of your organization in implementing these practices. Be aware, however, that this step cannot be addressed effectively until your organization has developed, implemented, and completed its strategy for becoming an HRO. **The metrics used by your organization to determine the success of its strategy for transforming into an HRO should be separate and distinct from the metrics used by your organization to determine the effectiveness of its HRO in sustaining high reliability operations.** In Chapter 3, we discussed the former—those steps and metrics associated with the critical strategic planning stage of the HRO journey; in this section, we suggest some broad-level metrics associated with sustaining each of the four HRO practices.

Keep in mind that metrics are tricky. The development of appropriate metrics is a difficult

Chapter 7 | **171**

skill to master. Many indicators that offer easy measurement—production rates, injury rates, the number of negative occurrences or events—are not useful to measure sustained HRO excellence. The metrics needed to ascertain that an organization is maintaining high reliability operations are based on continuous improvement. These metrics will be different for each HRO based on its industry, operations, and culture.

If the four HRO practices represent the desired end state of a HRO, then any measures of effective HRO operations must be oriented toward the success of implementing (and maintaining) these practices and the actions that support them. With that in mind, Table 7-1 provides some examples of metrics that could be used to measure success in implementing and sustaining each of the HRO practices. These are not industry-specific or all-inclusive, but rather are intended to help you develop metrics appropriate for your organization. Note also that there is overlap between the lines of inquiry and the suggested metrics—this is normal, as the metrics are typically an outgrowth of the lines of inquiry.

Lines of inquiry and the implementation and use of metrics should enable you to determine the success of your organization in aligning the various levels of your culture of reliability with the values that characterize an HRO. Depending on what you discover, you can investigate methods to help you better align your organization's culture of reliability with HRO practices or continue on in the same direction you are currently headed.

172 | High Reliability Operations • A Practical Guide to Avoid the System Accident

Table 7-1. Actions, Lines of Inquiry, and Suggested Metrics*

HRO Practice 1: Manage the System, not the Parts	
Associated Actions	**Lines of Inquiry**
Ensure Safety System Selected Provides Safety • Understand technical and operational underpinnings. • Verify the management system provides the safety and nothing else (positive control). • Understand the precepts of high reliability operations, the warning signs of system accidents, and the HRO programs used to avoid them. • Know how to evaluate the culture of reliability to assess HRO effectiveness.	• To what degree are documented annual performance objectives in line with espoused safety values? Consider the current operating efficiency of the plant (customer management alignment) • To what degree do strategic and tactical plans align with transparent operational goals (management–employee alignment)? • Are technical courses readily available to help managers understand the technical underpinnings of the business? • Are courses on high reliability theory, normal accident theory, and culture of reliability readily available? • What are the initial (baseline) and annual proficiency scores of managers in key technical positions? • Do you have an adequate number of managers with the appropriate technical education and/or experience to understand the technical underpinnings of the business? • How long do technically qualified managers typically remain in their jobs to gain technical proficiency? • How does the performance of managers compare to their technical proficiency and currency of training (compare number of incidences occurring within a manager's area relative to the number of opportunities for errors)? • Does management use a systematic process for planning, coordinating, and evaluating the safety impacts of decisions related to major changes in organizational structures and functions, leadership, policies, programs, and resources? • How committed is management to ensuring the safety system provides safety? To what extent are safety analysis reports for each hazardous operations: - Published and available? - Practical? - Readable? - Understandable?

Suggested Metrics

• Flow the objectives, measures, targets, and initiative from the transformation gap analysis and other strategic initiatives (Chapter 3) to annual performance evaluations for high- and mid-level managers.
- Measure the rate of completion of these initiatives (the progress made toward achieving the strategy and the staying power).

Chapter 7 | **173**

Table 7-1. Actions, Lines of Inquiry, and Suggested Metrics*

HRO Practice 1:
Manage the System, not the Parts

Associated Actions	Lines of Inquiry

Manage the Safety System to Reduce Variability
 	
• Develop and deploy safety system
• Stress the need to minimize consequences of hazardous operations.
   - Publish prioritized list of hazards to avoid.
   - Maintain focus on preventing system accidents at all costs and at all times (no reduction in focus or resources).
• Stress importance of staying within established safety system regardless of impact to production.
• Provide resources and infrastructure to ensure system remains effective.
• Insist on right technical talent with adequate training and expertise (detailed knowledge of equipment, processes, and systems).
• Evaluate the operation of the HRO system.
   - Look for common-mode failures.
   - Evaluate measures used to determine HRO sustainability.
	• How knowledgeable are employees about the safety system? How is the content of the safety analysis reports managed?
	
	• Are surveys made to determine how employees perceive managers? What do such surveys show with respect to the perceived visibility of the manager on the shop floor and about managers' understanding of the safety issues related to the work being performed?
	
	• Does your organization ensure that personnel, equipment, procedures, and other resources are available and adequate to assure safety?
	
	• Does your organization plan work appropriately by incorporating job-site conditions, organization structures, systems, and components, and human-system interfaces into its decisions?
	
	• How effectively does your organization use work planning and control?
	
	• Are complete, accurate, and up-to-date design documents such as as-builts, procedures, and work packages available?
	
	• Are facilities and equipment maintained in ready condition?
	
	• Are employees provided with procedures that actually work and provided the necessary level of protection (have employee demonstrate the use of the procedure to perform the work)?

Suggested Metrics

• Implement continuous improvement initiatives such as Lean management or Six Sigma to free resources for strategic initiatives.
   - Measure the rate of completion of these initiatives.
   - Measure the effectiveness of the initiatives over time (also measure whether the improvement was sustained).
• Use total productivity measures that consider human resources, energy expenditures, cash, and other resources in addition to product output.
• Measure downtime due to process, procedure, material, and equipment delays (a balanced system will not experience a high rate of down time due to production support systems).

continued

High Reliability Operations • A Practical Guide to Avoid the System Accident

Table 7-1. Actions, Lines of Inquiry, and Suggested Metrics*

HRO Practice 1:
Manage the System, not the Parts

Associated Actions	Lines of Inquiry

Foster a Culture of Reliability
• Provide the right training, tools, and support.
• Enable employees to make conservative decisions.
• Ensure proficiency through continuous hands-on work.
• Establish a culture of reliability.
  - Instill trust.
  - Encourage open questioning of and challenges to the safety system.
  - Monitor, evaluate, and use feedback to recharge efforts.
	• What percentage of employees are trained and proficient relative to the number required to maintain production rates?
	• Compare the requirements of the various critical job positions with the qualifications of those employees filling those positions.
	• What is the proficiency of the employees vs. the requirements of the jobs?
	• Does your organization have a policy prohibiting harassment and retaliation for raising safety concerns? Is this policy enforced?
	• Do employee behaviors and interactions encourage the free flow of information related to system safety issues and differing professional opinions? Are issues in the corrective action program identified and are self-assessments used regularly?
	• Do policies require and reinforce the idea that employees have both the right and the responsibility to raise system safety issues through all available means, including avenues outside their chain of command?
	• Do employees believe that managers are willing and able to solve safety issues?

Suggested Metrics
• Ensure the system of rewards and sanctions is aligned with the HRO practices by measuring the rate of noncompliance.

Model Organizational Learning • Involve employees in daily struggle to deal with conflicts between performance and safety. • Think through consequences for entire life-cycle before making decisions. • Demonstrate genuine desire to know the health of the business, good or bad, and to address the issues, not the symptoms.	• Are managers willing to openly dialog with employees about conflicts between production and safety? • Do managers walk the shop floor? • Is feedback used effectively to reduce the number of repeat occurrences, incidences, and events (issues management)? • How effective is the feedback system in identifying systemic issues and resolving them so they do not escalate? • How is information about the organization's culture of reliability collected and interpreted? Are actions taken by management if the culture indicates areas that need improvement? • What percentage of processes are modified based on learning from feedback (vs. the total number of processes implemented in a specified time period)?

Chapter 7   **175**

Table 7-1. Actions, Lines of Inquiry, and Suggested Metrics*

HRO Practice 1: Manage the System, not the Parts	
Associated Actions	**Lines of Inquiry**

• Evaluate work performance and the culture of reliability (managers and employees).
  - Obtain first-hand feedback from employees by routinely walking shop floors.
  - Use tracking and trending data to look for precursors to bigger problems.
  - Use Causal Factors Analysis process to investigate information-rich events.
  - Learn from others' mistakes.
• Adjust operations—effectively address causal factors to solve the root problem and measure effectiveness of corrective actions.
• Continually refine the safety system.
  - Continuously optimize processes and remove no-value added requirements.
	• Does your organization systematically collect, evaluate, and communicate relevant operating experience to affected stakeholders in a timely manner?
	• How many refinements have been made to the safety system? Have these refinements been effective?

Suggested Metrics

• Measure the rate of nonstrategic initiatives funded and implemented each fiscal year.

• Measure the rate of completion of strategic initiatives.

Table 7-1. Actions, Lines of Inquiry, and Suggested Metrics*

HRO Practice 2: Reduce System Variability	
Associated Actions	**Lines of Inquiry**

Deploy Break-the-Chain Safety Framework
• Reduce interactive complexity and coupling of system.
• Reduce physical hazard using increased rigor proportional to level of consequence.
• Fully implement and use Human Performance Improvement (HPI+) framework.
  - Recognize, identify, and act to minimize human error precursors.
  - Recognize error modes of employees to minimize most error prone flaws.
• Deploy independent redundant barriers to mitigate consequences using increased rigor proportional to level of consequence.
  - Challenge complacency.
  - Provide incentives for staff to identify flaws in standard operating procedures.
	• How many repeat findings are discovered through start-up readiness reviews, repeat occurrences, incidences, and events?
	• How many errors or failures are not detected until an event investigation occurs?
	• How effective is work planning in identifying all work hazards (evaluate by comparing hazards identified in planning packages vs. those found by the workforce vs. those discovered in events)?
	• What percentage of pre-work briefs review human performance error precursors?
	• What percentage of post-work reviews compare work-as-imagined vs. work-as-done with regards to detected human error precursors (to provide immediate feedback)?
	• How many human performance error precursors are observed? Has this number been reduced over time?
	• How many pre-work briefs review safety barrier viability before work is begun?
	• What percentage of post-work reviews compare work-as-imagined vs. work-as-done relative to weak or missing barriers (to provide immediate feedback)?
	• How many missing or flawed barriers are observed? Has this number changed over time?
	• Does your organization communicate human error prevention techniques through pre-work briefs, peer checking, and proper documentation of work?
	• To what degree is the safety management process known and used by the workforce in everyday work?

Suggested Metrics
• Establish process capability for production lines—use control charts to detect process drift.

Chapter 7 | **177**

Table 7-1. Actions, Lines of Inquiry, and Suggested Metrics*

HRO Practice 2: Reduce System Variability	
Associated Actions	**Lines of Inquiry**
Evaluate the Operation of the Safety System • Measure and minimize gap between work-as-imagined and work-as-done. • Be vigilant for common operational pitfalls. • Evaluate operations using specific indicators and measures.	• Are employees supplied with procedures that actually work and provide the necessary level of protection (have the employee demonstrate the use of the procedure to perform the work)? • To what degree are procedures followed for all operations (technical and administrative), as evidenced by observations that the procedures are visible and actively read by the operator? • To what degree and consistency are human performance error precursors and barriers considered in prework discussions? • What is the consistency and quality of prework briefs? Do they include physical walk downs while the planned work is being discussed? • Observe the existence and use of administrative and engineering controls. • Observe the proper selection and use of personal protective equipment (PPE). • Observe the proper use of warning/caution signs (displayed while the hazard is present and removed when hazard is removed to reduce complacency). • Are assessments of sufficient depth? That is, are they comprehensive, objective, and self-critical? • Does your organization periodically assess the effectiveness of oversight programs? - Do self-assessments and management assessments adequately identify problems before they reach the event stage?

Suggested Metrics

• Evaluate the effectiveness of work planning and control.
  - Measure the rate of errors found in the field (work-as-imagined vs. work-as-done).
  - Measure the rate of process deviations.
  - Measure the rate of schedule non-compliance for production and projects.
  - Measure the rate of terminated/cancelled/deferred jobs.
  - Measure the rate of errors or failures detected by an event or incident (includes procedure non-adherence).
• Establish a rate for HPI+ precursors from incidents, accidents, assessments, and lessons learned. Measure the reduction rate of HPI+ precursors.

continued

Table 7-1. Actions, Lines of Inquiry, and Suggested Metrics*

HRO Practice 2: Reduce System Variability	
Associated Actions	**Lines of Inquiry**

Suggested Metrics

- Use employee safety measures such as:
  - Lost time accidents
  - Total recordable cases
  - First aid
- Establish a rate for technical safety requirement violations.
  - Measure the rate of violations.
  - Measure the incidence of new information.
  - Determine equipment and facility reliability.
  - Measure production downtime caused by facility or equipment.
  - Measure rate of preventive maintenance performed within the grace period.
  - Measure deferred maintenance backlog.
  - Measure corrective maintenance backlog.
- Establish risk triggers for Break-the-Chain defenses-in-depth.
  - Measure the rate at which risk triggers are tripped.
  - Measure the rate the same risk trigger is tripped (i.e., repeat occurrences).
  - Measure the rate risk triggers are tripped and then investigated (or not).
- Determine project management health.
  - Measure cost performance index (CPI).
  - Measure schedule performance index (SPI).

Associated Actions	Lines of Inquiry
Systematically Adjust Processes • Revise individual process procedures based on small failures. • Implement effective corrective actions. • Learn lessons. • Verify corrective measures provide desired change.	• How effective is your organization's operating experience program (evaluate the number and quality of changes to procedures, equipment, and training programs)? • Is your corrective action tracking system effective (is implementation verified and evaluated to be effective before closeout is completed)? • Is your organization willing to follow through thoroughly with all corrective actions identified in assessments and causal analysis investigations?

Chapter 7 | **179**

Table 7-1. Actions, Lines of Inquiry, and Suggested Metrics*

HRO Practice 3: Foster a Culture of Reliability	
Associated Actions	**Lines of Inquiry**
Enable Employees to Make Conservative Decisions • Provide effective, continuous technical education to increase understanding of key technical systems for operations and safety. • Provide effective, continuous education on safety culture, organizational learning, and conservative decision-making fundamentals to provide the basis for conservative decisions. • Provide effective, continuous, hands-on training to ensure decisions are founded on real-life physical processes. • Ensure infrastructure supports employees in maintaining positive control of their work environment. • Provide flexible and adaptable organizational structures appropriate for operational challenges.	• Are technical courses available to help employees understand the technical underpinnings of the business? • Are courses on high reliability theory, normal accident theory, and safety culture available? • Does your organization provide adequate training and knowledge transfer to ensure technical competency? • How effective is training within your organization? • How do the initial (baseline) scores of employees in key technical positions compare to their annual proficiency scores? • What percentage of employees are certified before work is begun? • What percentage of employees maintain job currency? • Does your organization use simulated work scenarios (or hands-on training) to evaluate employees' ability to make proper time-critical decisions? • Observe the level of ownership of the organization's process. • Observe how knowledgeable the employees are of the barriers put in place to protect them and their co-workers. • Does management maintain accountability for important safety decisions with systems and sanctions? Is this aligned with safety policies? Does management reinforce behaviors and outcomes that reflect safety as an overriding priority? • Do employees use a systematic process to make risk-significant decisions by formally defining, communicating, and implementing decision authority? • Do employees use conservative assumptions and require demonstration that a proposed action is safe? • Is there a stop work program that is enforced when operational safety is uncertain?

Suggested Metrics

• Map the following (establish a baseline) to errors:
   - Pre-work briefings
   - Pre-work inspection/walk-down
   - Management walk downs
   - Post-work lessons learned
• Measure the rate of improvement with increased discipline in pre-work briefs and walk downs and post-work briefs relative to supervisor presence at the job site.

continued

180   High Reliability Operations • A Practical Guide to Avoid the System Accident

Table 7-1. Actions, Lines of Inquiry, and Suggested Metrics*

HRO Practice 3: Foster a Culture of Reliability	
Associated Actions	**Lines of Inquiry**
Ensure Proficiency Through Hands-On Work • Reduce process inefficiencies to provide more time to perform hands-on work to retain proficiency. • Require proof of task proficiency before work is initiated.	• What degree of employee downtime is due to process or equipment delays? • What is the error rate of employees vs. the opportunities for errors to evaluate the effectiveness of training. • Are employees evaluated using simulated work scenarios (or hands-on training) to determine their current level of proficiency vs. that obtained in initial training?

Suggested Metrics

• Measure the rate of incidents, accidents, and events reported by employees.

• Measure the rates at which employees pass drills and simulations.

Encourage Open Questioning of and Challenges to the Safety System • Managers walk the talk and transparently demonstrate espoused cultural values. • Employees challenge unsafe or unclear operations and openly communicate issues to supervisors. • Supervisors appropriately act on issues raised by employees and provide feedback on resolution. • All employees share openly without fear of retribution to build mindfulness and enable swift learning with the focus on finding cures for problems rather than prevention. • Line supervisors provide immediate feedback on decisions to keep errors small, to keep the system safely operating, and to retain resilience.	• To what degree is the workforce knowledgeable of the safety system? Do employees believe in it? • Are work area culture surveys made to evaluate the willingness and ability of employees to implement the HRO safety system? • Do employees use simulated work scenarios (or hands-on training) to evaluate their ability to make conservative decisions? • How effective are classes on conservative decision making (as determined by employee-supervisor feedback during post-work reviews)? • Are work area surveys used to evaluate the willingness and ability of employees to make conservative decisions? • Do employees question their assigned work? To what degree? • Are employees able and willing to recognize and report events? • Do surveys indicate that employees are willing to challenge problems? Are they satisfied their voices are heard? • Does the work environment allow and encourage employees to raise concerns to managers, customers, or external regulators without fear of retaliation? • Do employees believe that harassment and retaliation for raising safety concerns will not be tolerated? • Are issues that could impact the system safety promptly identified and fully evaluated? Are timely actions taken that are commensurate with the significance of these issues? • Does your organization implement corrective actions with a low threshold for identifying issues?

Chapter 7   **181**

Table 7-1. Actions, Lines of Inquiry, and Suggested Metrics*

HRO Practice 3: Foster a Culture of Reliability	
Associated Actions	**Lines of Inquiry**

Suggested Metrics

- Survey the culture with respect to HRO attributes. Determine the willingness of employees to identify problems without fear of retribution.

- Measure the rate of approved and implemented employee-generated improvement initiatives.

- Determine the success of resolution of differing professional opinions. Survey employees who hold differing professional opinions and determine their satisfaction with the outcome of the situation.

Table 7-1. Actions, Lines of Inquiry, and Suggested Metrics*

HRO Practice 4: Learn and Adapt as an Organization	
Associated Actions	**Lines of Inquiry**

Generate Decision-Making Information
 	
• Use a tiered approach to organizational feedback based on the significance of the process and data.
  - Tier 0: Program start up
  - Tier 1: Daily supervisor-employee feedback
  - Tier 2: Tracking and trending
  - Tier 3: Event investigation
  - Tier 4: Learning from external events and benchmarking
• Integrate and interpret feedback data to enable better decision making.
  - Evaluate organizational significance.
  - Extrapolate singular event data to the organizational level.
  - Compare results between system events to discover cycles.
  - Evaluate the effectiveness of the HRO practices.
	• To what degree is each tier of feedback used in your organization?
	• How effective is each feedback tier in identifying and resolving problems in the system?
	• Does your management effectively review collective reports to look for negative trends or safety culture issues that could indicate a problem with safety?
	• To what degree is an operating experience program (lessons learned from other industry system accidents) read and used by employees and managers in everyday work planning?
	• Does your organization implement and institutionalize operating experience as evidenced by changes to procedures, equipment, and training programs?
	• How many repeat findings are identified through start-up readiness reviews, repeat occurrences, incidences, and events?

Suggested Metrics

• Ensure the availability of knowledge capture through the use of performance metrics and trends.

Refine the HRO System: Apply a System Approach to Reduce Variability • Characterize the organization's culture of reliability. • Deploy Six Sigma and Lean techniques to continually optimize the system to provide more time for safety. • Improve training based on effectiveness to modify employee behavior.	• How many Six Sigma improvement projects have been undertaken to optimize existing safety systems? • How effective are these Six Sigma improvement projects (characterized by reduction in overall process steps and time)? • Does the behavior of employees indicate change after a lesson learned is issued?

continued

Chapter 7 | **183**

Table 7-1. Actions, Lines of Inquiry, and Suggested Metrics*

HRO Practice 4: Learn and Adapt as an Organization	
Associated Actions	**Lines of Inquiry**

Suggested Metrics

- Measure the rate of recommendations not implemented from:
  - Readiness reviews
  - Internal audits
  - Management self assessments
  - CFA investigations (latent organizational weaknesses)
  - Other event or incident investigations
  - Drills and simulations
  - Actual errors in the field versus test results from training
  - Lessons learned internally and externally
- Measure the rate of repeat findings (i.e., corrective actions that fail to fix the problem) from:
  - Readiness reviews
  - Internal audits
  - Management self assessments
  - CFA investigations (latent organizational weaknesses)
  - Other event or incident investigations
  - Drills and simulations
  - Actual errors in the field versus test results from training
  - Lessons learned internally and externally
  - Other event or incident investigations
  - Drills and simulations
  - Actual errors in the field vs. test results from training
  - Lessons learned internally and externally

*The content of this table adapted from information found in Corcoran, 2007a and NRC, 2006 with additional entries developed specifically for the HRO practices.

What If My Organization's Culture Is Not Healthy?

If, after much consternation, you decide you do not like what the results of the culture evaluation show, you have two options. First, you can modify your approach to the HRO practice or practices that do not seem to be effective and try again. Alternately, your organization can hire a consultant who specializes in organizational culture modification to help you institute long-term fixes. Information about each approach is provided in the following sections.

The Simple Fix: Modify and Reapply the Target HRO Practice

The lines of inquiry introduced in Table 7-1 are arranged by HRO practice (and associated action); this was done to help you identify specific actions that may not be effective within your organization. If you note that your organization is not succeeding in a particular area, the first course of business is to modify the programs associated with that HRO practice or associated action and try again. This is not a cop-out or a simple accommodational fix; many consultants in the field of organizational culture recommend this approach. For example, Edgar Schein (1999) counsels organizations to attempt to change culture only when there is a specific problem to be solved, and only when they can work with existing cultural strengths:

> *"Never start with the idea of changing culture. Always start with the issue the organization faces; only when those business issues are clear should you ask yourself whether the culture aids or hinders resolving the issues. Always think initially of the culture as your source of strength. It is the residue of your past successes. Even if some elements of the culture look dysfunctional, remember that they are*

probably only a few among a large set of others that continue to be strengths. If changes need to be made in how the organization is run, try to build on existing cultural strengths rather than attempting to change those elements that may be weaknesses" (Schein, 1999, p. 189).

The intent of the simple fix is to focus on modifying the HRO programs to fit your culture while still obtaining the required level of safety. Typically, this is much easier than trying to change your organization's culture. Attempting to modify the culture or behavior of an entire organization is a long, arduous, and often overwhelming challenge.

Long-term Fix: Find a Good Consultant

If you determine that your organizational culture must be changed to ensure safe and reliable operations, be prepared for a struggle. Cultural change is hard, slow, and subject to frequent relapse. Even so, there are steps an organization can take to nudge its culture toward greater mindfulness (Weick and Sutcliffe, 2001):

- Exercise vigilance in tracking down bad news, stalking the anomalous, and requiring proof of safety and reliability.

- Clearly define and explain terms such as "information-rich event," "near-miss," "anomalous occurrence," and "culture of reliability."

- Make your culture work for you: use the power of social influence, understand how feedback is used, use symbols to clarify and crystallize principles, and exercise control through your culture of reliability.

> **The leader's role is to:**
>
> - Define reality: where we are today.
>
> - Define the vision: where we want to be.
>
> - Define how to get there.
>
> You then need to know what characteristics and attributes you want to see in the workplace, and what you want the culture to achieve.
>
> *(Persson, p. 19)*

- Encourage cultural change by acting your way into new values. Demonstrate that safety comes first.

- Monitor and respect the health and strength of your culture. Keep your finger on the pulse and admire and encourage the natural resilience of the culture. But don't be surprised when attempted changes inspire guerilla warfare.

If you come to the realization that your organization's culture is truly unhealthy, you probably need to get outside professional help. Although there are many good sources of information that will help you gain an understanding of what must be done, you should probably enlist the professional services of an outside consultant. Such a consultant should have a proven track record in facilitating the process of cultural change. Make sure the consultant is a good fit for your organization and then commit to the long haul—there are no short-term fixes for this type of organizational change.

Chapter 8

Chapter 8

Wrapping it Up: What You Should Take Away from this Guide

This chapter answers the following questions:

- How does Deming's Theory of Profound Knowledge (1994) support and inform the four HRO practices?

- Are the four HRO practices distinct or interrelated?

- How does an organization begin the HRO transformation process?

- How does an organization sustain high reliability operations?

- What "pearls of wisdom" can I take away from this guide to help me in my day-to-day management of an HRO?

You have just completed a quick tour of the practices—and pitfalls—associated with HROs. If you have taken the time to read this guide, your organization is likely one that cannot face or recover from the consequences of a system accident. Your first decision is whether or not to proceed down the path that leads to high reliability operations.

We've tried to provide tools and examples that will help you with that decision—and with the steps you should follow if you decide to go forward. The material we have presented, developed from the research of many individuals, spans the subjects of high reliability, normal accident theory, safety culture, organizational accidents, human error, and other relevant topics. We provide Table 7-1 as a summary of the complete HRO process described in this text along with recommended lines of inquiry and metrics for each HRO practice. The main sources we have used are indicated in the reference list; we encourage you to read and study these source materials.

Our intent in this guide was to interpret, integrate, and apply existing concepts about systems and high reliability operations to the day-to-day work of high-hazard operations. We believe we have developed some tools that provide practical and realistic approaches to attaining and sustaining high reliability operations. However, because every industry and organization is different, we also believe these tools and approaches should be adapted to fit your specific needs. The material we have presented is intended as a foundation for those of you who plan to begin or continue the quest to become an HRO; it can also be helpful to those interested in applying and understanding the results of the Causal Factors Analysis process, which is further described in *Causal Factors Analysis: An Approach for Organizational Learning* (Hartley et al., 2008).

In this chapter, we aim to summarize the key points of this guide and leave you with a few pointers that can help make your HRO journey smoother and more successful.

The Importance of a System Approach
Many existing texts describe the attributes of an HRO, most of which were gleaned from organizational studies of high-hazard industries with good safety records. Although these

Chapter 8 **189**

attributes are useful, we were interested in developing practices that are directly related to the physics of safety, and we wanted to develop an HRO safety system that was rooted in systems theory. The result is our Break-the-Chain Framework, which is a physics-based safety system that is grounded in Deming's Theory of Profound Knowledge (1994). The relationships between the major components of Deming's Theory of Profound Knowledge and our four HRO practices developed for this text are presented in Table 8-1.

Table 8-1. Relationship Between Deming's Theory of Profound Knowledge and the Four HRO Practices	
Element of Deming's Theory of Profound Knowledge*	**HRO Practice**
Knowledge of (and appreciation for) a system. A system is a network of interdependent components working together to accomplish a specific aim. Systems must be managed, as they tend to perpetuate their own goals and resist change. The greater the interdependence between components, the greater the need for communication and cooperation among these components and the greater the need for overall management. Failure of management to comprehend the interdependence between components can be the cause of loss. The efforts of the various divisions in a company, each given a job, are not additive but interdependent. Each component part is obligated to contribute its best to the system rather than maximize its own profit, and may even operate at a loss in order to optimize the entire system.	**Manage the system, not the parts.** This practice focuses on, and must be implemented by, managers. Systems, while providing powerful defenses to protect against catastrophic accidents, also present a new set of challenges to managers. The manager must ensure the system provides the requisite level of safety and doesn't introduce more significant failure mechanisms with other consequences. The manager must oversee the development and deployment of the system and the manager must drive to obtain accurate, timely, and continuous feedback on the health of the system. The manager must be courageous enough to persevere even when initiatives are difficult to implement and measure, and must communicate a strong commitment to safety and reliability through both actions and words. The manager must foster a culture of reliability in which open and honest communications are expected and acted upon, which results in continuous organizational learning and adapting.

continued

Table 8-1. Relationship Between Deming's Theory of Profound Knowledge and the Four HRO Practices

Element of Deming's Theory of Profound Knowledge*	HRO Practice
Knowledge of variation. Organizational systems are highly variable. Organizations can deal with variability by first measuring and then comparing predictions vs. performance. Knowledge about the different sources of uncertainty should be used to refine the system or process being implemented (i.e. reduce variability). Measurement is an iterative process; it is not to be performed just once.	**Reduce system variability.** To function as an HRO, an organization must deploy a robust HRO system, evaluate the performance of the system, and continuously reduce performance variability to decrease the likelihood of unexpected system events. The HRO system introduced in this text consists of six steps in the Break-the-Chain Framework. Variability is reduced in the Break-the-Chain Framework by minimizing hazards, reducing the negative influences of complex interactivity and tight coupling, minimizing human error, and explicitly using redundant independent barriers as backups in case other actions fail.
Knowledge of psychology. A leader of transformation must learn and understand the psychology of individuals, the psychology of a group (commonly called the culture of the organization), and the psychology of change. Psychology helps managers understand people, the interaction between people and circumstances, the interaction between customer and supplier, and the interaction between managers, employees, and any system of management.	**Foster a strong culture of reliability.** Because no system works unless it is used, managers want their employees to fully implement, believe, and police the use of the HRO system. Because no system is perfect, managers want their employees to challenge the system and bring shortcomings to the surface before incidents occur. We use the term culture of reliability to indicate an organizational culture that focuses not only on safety, but on consistent, dependable, and excellent products and services. A culture of reliability, according to our definition, encompasses: • Employees who are trained and empowered to make conservative decisions on the shop-floor. • Employees who retain their proficiency through continuous hands-on work. • An organization (managers and employees) that daily demonstrates a culture of reliability by transparently walking the talk and challenging and acting to correct unsafe conditions to protect against the system accident.

Chapter 8 | 191

Table 8-1. Relationship Between Deming's Theory of Profound Knowledge and the Four HRO Practices

Element of Deming's Theory of Profound Knowledge*	HRO Practice
Knowledge of knowledge (theory of knowledge). Management in any form is prediction. Managers predict future outcome, with the risk of being wrong, based on observations of the past. Rational prediction builds knowledge through the systematic revision and extension of theoretical principles; such revision is based on a comparison of prediction and observation. Feedback helps validate, improve, or invalidate the theory. Without theory, there is no learning. It is only in a state of statistical control that statistical theory provides, with a high degree of belief, prediction of performance in the immediate future. Information, no matter how complete and immediate, is not knowledge. Knowledge has temporal spread and develops from the testing of theory. Without a theory against which to test the information, there is no way to use information received at a specific point in time.	**Learn and adapt as an organization.** HROs cannot survive solely on the basis of safety statistics. HROs must be learning organizations and strive for excellence through continuous organizational renewal. Because safety is a top priority for HROs, the aim is to gather as much relevant information as possible and turn it into knowledge to stimulate organizational learning. We provide a tiered approach to organizational learning that provides feedback from start-up processes, daily supervisor-employee interactions, tracking and trending of data, causal factors analysis, and learning from external lessons. To encourage learning, we can work our way through the Break-the-Chain Framework in reverse to help understand where the safety system is weak and thus to continuously refine the HRO system.

*Deming, 1994

Deming's theory (1994) allowed us to roll up the HRO practices to a more fundamental level. That is, we were able to understand and explain the why behind the what. This allows our HRO practices to be adapted for any industry or organization.

As with the elements of Deming's theory, our HRO practices and their associated actions are integrated and interrelated. Because of this, the separate presentation of these practices in this guide is somewhat artificial, although useful for explaining the concepts. In reality, neither the concepts nor the practices can be entirely separated; don't frustrate yourself in an effort to compartmentalize the practices or the actions or metrics associated with them.

To become an HRO, you must first understand what an HRO is, then you must develop a plan that ensures that you have the resources and commitment of the entire management team to help you achieve HRO status. To aid in this endeavor, we provided guidance and examples about how to become an HRO through the use of seven elements (from the McKinsey 7S approach, first published by Thomas J. Peters and Robert H. Waterman in 1982) in conjunction with the four HRO practices. We recommend using the 7S elements to drive your strategy to close gaps between current and desired performance, and to develop measures of effectiveness to ascertain how well the transformation is going.

Unfortunately, as hard as it is becoming an HRO, sustaining high reliability operations on an ongoing basis is even harder. The problem is that maintaining a high state of readiness and chronic unease goes against almost every human tendency. A substantial amount of time and effort will have to be pumped into the system on a daily basis to counter the human tendency toward complacency. To be successful, you need to help your organization develop and implement a safety system and then ensure that you and your employees stick to it religiously.

Pointers to Help You Achieve and Maintain High Reliability Operations

Many important concepts, based on the research of others, have been presented in this guide (Table 7-1 provides a convenient summary). For example, the concepts of Weick and Sutcliffe (2001) regarding a mindful approach to high reliability operations (Chapter 2) are key to the long-term sustainability of an HRO. We realize, however, that you, as a busy manager, may appreciate some simple "pearls of wisdom" to help you in your daily management of an HRO. Here's our quick list for you:

- Manage from the shop floor, not the office.

- Remember, it can happen here. Focus on the physics—it isn't what you think, it's what is.

- Maintain chronic unease—question and verify everything.

- Trust permeates all aspects of work. Walk the talk; make sure your underlying assumptions match your espoused values.

- Break that chain between threat and hazard!

- A culture of reliability sustains an HRO; an unhealthy culture inhibits an HRO.

References

ACSNI, *Organising for Safety: Third Report of the ACSNI (Advisory Committee on the Safety of Nuclear Installations) Study Group on Human Factors*, Health and Safety Commission (of Great Britain), HSE Books, Sudbury, England, 1993.

Anderson, V., and L. Johnson, *Systems Thinking Basics: From Concepts to Causal Loops*, Pegasus Communications, Inc. Waltham, MA, 1997.

CAIB (Columbia Accident Investigation Board), *Columbia Accident Investigation Board Final Report, Vol. 1*, August 2003.

Corcoran, William R., 2007a. *Safety Culture - Back to the Basics, Version 12.03*, NSRC Corporation, August 2007.

Corcoran, William R., 2007b. *The Phoenix Handbook*, NRSC Corporation, 2007.

Corcoran, William R., 2007d. Private Communication with Rick Hartley, 2007.

Dekker, Sidney, *The Field Guide to Understanding Human Error*, Ashgate Publishing Limited, Aldershot, UK, 2006.

Defense Science Board Permanent Task Force on Nuclear Weapons Surety, *Report on the Unauthorized Movement of Nuclear Weapons*, Office of Undersecretary of Defense for Acquisition, Technology, and Logistics, Washington DC, Ch. 1, p. 20301-3140, February 2008, Revised April 2008.

Deming, W. Edwards,*The New Economics for Industry*, Government, Education, Massachusetts Institute of Technology, Center for Advanced Engineering Study, Cambridge, 1994.

EFCOG (Energy Facilities Contractor Operating Group), *Task Group on Safety Culture*, (adapted from the Institute of Nuclear Power Operations), June 2008.

Greenleaf, R. K., Servant Leadership: *A Journey Into the Nature of Legitimate Power and Greatness,* Paulist Press, Mahwah, NJ, 1977.

Grenoble, Dr. Skip, In: Blanchard, Dave, *Logistically Speaking: The Trouble with Benchmarking*, May 2005 <http://outsourced-logistics.com/operations_strategy/outlog_story_7206/indexl.html>, accessed in June 2008.

Hartley, Richard S., Dan J. Swaim, and William R. Corcoran, *Causal Factors Analysis: An Approach for Organizational Learning*, Babcock & Wilcox Technical Services Pantex LLC (B&W Pantex), 2008.

Hopkins, A., 2002, *Safety Culture, Mindfulness, and Safe Behaviour: Converging Ideas?* Working Paper 7, National Centre for OHS Regulation, Australian National University, December 2002 <http://www.ohs.anu.edu.au/publications/pdf/*wp%207%20-%20Hopkins.pdf*>, accessed in May 2008.

Hopkins, A., 2006a, *A Corporate Dilemma: To Be a Learning Organisation or to Minimise Liability*, Working Paper 43, National Centre for OHS Regulation, Australian National University, January 2006, <http://www.ohs.anu.edu.au/publications/pdf/wp%2043%20-%20Hopkins.pdf>, accessed in May 2008.

Hopkins, A.., 2006b, *Studying Organisational Cultures and Their Effects on Safety,* Working Paper 44, National Centre for OHS Regulation, Australian National University, May 2006, <http://www.ohs.anu.edu.au/publications/pdf/*wp%2044%20-%20Hopkins.pdf*>, accessed in May 2008.

Hopkins, A., 2006c, *Holding Corporate Leaders Responsible*, Working Paper 48, National Centre for OHS Regulation, Australian National University, August 2006, <http://www.ohs.anu.edu.au/publications/pdf/*wp%2048%20-%20Hopkins.pdf*>, accessed in May 2008.

Hopkins, A., 2006d, *What Are We to Make of Safe Behaviour Programs?* Safety Science, Vol. 44, No.77, 2006, pp. 583–597.

Hopkins, A., 2007,*The Problem of Defining High Reliability Organisations*, Working Paper 51, National Centre for OHS Regulation, Australian National University, January 2007, <http://www.ohs.anu.edu.au/publications/pdf/wp%2051%20-%20Hopkins.pdf>, accessed in May 2008.

Hopkins, A., *Thinking About Process Safety Indicators,* Working Paper 53, National Centre for OHS Regulation , Australian National University, May 2007, <http://www.ohs.anu.edu.au/publications/pdf/*wp%2053%20-%20Hopkins.pdf*>, accessed in May 2008.

Hopkins, A., *Identifying and Responding to Warnings: The Case of Australia's Air Traffic Control Organisations,* Working Paper 57, National Centre for OHS Regulation, Australian National University, June 2007, <http://www.ohs.anu.edu.au/publications/pdf/wp%2057%20-%20Hopkins.pdf>, accessed in May 2008.

INSAG (International Nuclear Safety Group), *Summary Report on the Post-Accident Review Meeting on the Chernobyl Accident*, INSAG-1, 1986.

INPO (Institute of Nuclear Power Operations), *Human Performance Fundamentals Course Reference*, December 2002.

INPO, (Institute of Nuclear Power Operations), *Human Performance Reference Manual*, INPO 06-003, 2006.

INPO, (Institute of Nuclear Power Operations), *Principles for a Strong Nuclear Safety Culture*, November 2004.

Kaplan, Robert S., and David P. Norton, *The Strategy Focused Organization: How Balanced Scorecard Companies Thrive in the New Business Environment*, Harvard Business School Press, Boston, 2001.

LaPorte, Todd R., and Paula M. Consolini, *Working in Practice But Not in Theory: Theoretical Challenges of High Reliability Organizations*, Journal of Public Administration Research and Theory, Vol. 1, No. 1, January 1991, pp. 19–48.

Lewis, Clarence Irving, *Mind and the World Order: An Outline of a Theory of Knowledge*, Charles Scribner's Sons, New York, 1929.

Marais, Karen, Nicolas Dulac,, and Nancy Levenson, *Beyond Normal Accidents and High Reliability Organizations: The Need for an Alternative Approach to Safety in Complex Systems*, March 24, 2004.

Mittelstaedt, Robert E. Jr., *Will Your Next Mistake be Fatal?*, Wharton School of Publishing, 2005.

Neuman, Johanna, FAA's *Culture of Coziness' Targeted in Airline Safety Hearing*, April 2008, <http://articles.latimes.com/2008/apr/04/business/fi-airlines4>, accessed in June 2008.

Nielson, Ron, Fear of Flying, <http://www.fearlessflight.com/*airplane-disasters-plane-crash-statistics*> (accessed in May 2008).

NRC (Nuclear Regulatory Commission), Issue Summary, 2006–13, ML061880341, *Information on the Changes Made to the Reactor Oversight Process to More Fully Address Safety Culture*, Office of Enforcement, U.S. Nuclear Regulatory Agency, Washington DC, July 31, 2006.

Perrow, Charles, Normal Accidents—*Living with High-Risk Technologies*, Princeton University Press, 1999.

Persson, Kertstin Dahlgren, *IAEA Safety Standards on Management Systems and Safety Culture,* International Atomic Energy Agency, Department of Nuclear Energy, Vienna, Austria.

Peters, Thomas J., and Robert H. Waterman, Jr., *In Search of Excellence*, Warner Books Inc., 1982.

Reason, James, *Human Error*, Ashgate Publishing Limited, Hants, England, 1990.

Reason, James, *Managing the Risk of Organizational Accidents*, Ashgate Publishing Limited, Hants, England, 1997.

Reason, James, *Achieving a Safe Culture: Theory and Practice,* Work and Stress, Issue 12, No. 3, 1998, pp. 293–306.

Rickover U.S.N., Admiral Hyman G., *Basic Principles for Doing Your Job*, (excerpts from a speech given to the Order of 5-48).

Roberts, Karlene H, *HRO Has Prominent History,* Anesthesia Patient Safety Foundation Newsletter, Vol. 18, No. 1, Spring 2003, pp. 1-16.

Sagan, Scott D., *The Limits of Safety,* Princeton University Press, Princeton, NJ, 1993.

Schein, Edgar, *Organizational Culture and Leadership,* 2nd ed., Jossey-Bass, San Francisco, CA, 1992.

Schein, Edgar, *The Corporate Culture Survival Guide,* Jossey-Bass, San Francisco, CA, 1999.

Schein, Edgar, *Organization Culture and Leadership,* 3rd ed., Wiley Publishers, NY, 2004.

Schein, Edgar, *Safety Culture Management in High Reliability Organizations*, (obtained from Dave Collins, Dominion Nuclear, July 2007).

Shewart, Walter, *Statistical Methods from the Viewpoint of Quality Control*, Graduate School of the Department of Agriculture, Washington, DC, 1939.

Turner, Barry A., and Nick F. Pidgeon, *Man-Made Disasters,* Butterworth-Heinemann, London,1997.

TXU (Texas Utilities), The Texas Utilities (now Luminant) *Causal Analysis Handbook,* Rev. 7, June 28, 2005.

U.S. DOE (U.S. Department of Energy), Order 5480.19, *Conduct of Operations Requirements for DOE Facilities,* Ch. 3.

U.S. DOE (U.S. Department of Energy), *Integrated Safety Management Manual,* 450.4-1, 2006.

U.S. DOE (U.S. Department of Energy), *Human Performance Handbook, Human Performance Improvement Concepts and Principles,* 2007.

von Bertalanffy, Ludwig, *General Systems Theory, Foundations, Development, Applications,* George Braziller, New York, 1968.

Weick, Karl and Sutcliffe, Kathleen, *Managing the Unexpected,* Jossey-Bass, A Wiley Company, 2001.

Weick, K. E., 2004. *Normal Accident Theory As Frame, Link, And Provocation,* Organizational Environment, 17, 1, 2004, pp. 27-31.

Wickens, Christopher D., *Engineering Psychology and Human Performance,* 2nd ed., Harper-Collins, 1992.

Wikipedia contributors, *Common Mode Failure,* October 20, 2007, <http://en.wikipedia.org/w/index.php?title=*Common_mode_failure&oldid=165847301*>, accessed in May 2008.

Wikipedia contributors, *Boiling Frog,* May 30, 2008, <http://en.wikipedia.org/w/index.php?title=*Boiling_frog&oldid=216018354*>, accessed 3 June 2008.

Zebroski, Edwin L., *Attributes of Seven Major Accidents,* Presented at American Nuclear Society Meeting, San Diego, June 2, 2003.

Notes

[1] Other major researchers on high reliability theory who have helped shape our views include K. Weick and K. Sutcliffe (2001) at the University of Michigan; S. Sagan (1993), a critic of HRO theory at Stanford; J. Reason (1990, 1997, 1998) at Manchester; and Charles Perrow (1999).

[2] Deming introduced the Theory of Profound Knowledge in his book *The New Economics* (1994). He was greatly influenced by the work of Ludwig von Bertalanffy (1968) and C.L. Lewis (1929) on system theory and by Walter Shewhart (1939) on statistical process control. His Theory of Profound Knowledge was a synthesis of this previous research and was provided as a primer to help managers understand their organizations and consequently make better decisions. The Theory of Profound Knowledge is arguably Deming's greatest work, yet he is better known for his application of statistical process control and continuous improvement.

[3] The design of safety programs needs to be done in partnership with other programs (administrative, policies, training, etc.). New policies or procedures should be questions while in design. Ask "what could be the unintended consequences of this change?" The organizational system must always be viewed as a whole and not just as a sum of its parts.

[4] We use the term safety system figuratively in this text. There is in reality no such thing as a safety system. Rather it is an aggregate of engineered safety, safety basis, administrative processes, operating policies, and organizational culture that taken collectively represents a safety envelope.

[5] The Causal Factors Analysis tool, as described further in Chapter 6 and the companion to this volume, *Causal Factors Analysis: An Approach to Organizational Learning*, (Hartley et al., 2008) is a good tool for this. CFA can help discover the systematic causes of events or incidents; also, when different CFA reports for different events are compared, it can help highlight event trends.

[6] Diane Vaughan developed this term based on her study of the O-ring failures in the Challenger accident. In this accident, "the range of expected error enlarged from the judgment that it was normal to have heat on the primary O-ring, to normal to have erosion on the primary O-ring, to normal to have gas blowby, to normal to have blowby reaching the

secondary O-ring, and finally to the judgment that it was normal to have erosion on the secondary O-ring" (CAIB 2003, p. 196).

[7] There is a difference in the use of the terms of violation and error. An error is a human action that unintentionally departs from an expected behavior. A violation, on the other hand, involves a deliberate deviation from an expected behavior or an intentional circumvention of known rules and policies. Whereas errors arise from the under-specification of various mental operations, many violations are created by procedural over-specification.

[8] The concept and idea of naming the Break-the-Chain Framework presented in this text was adapted from *Will Your Next Mistake be Fatal?* by Robert Mittelstaedt, Wharton School Publishing, 2005.

[9] More detail about how these tools are used in CFA investigations can be found in the companion volume to this guide, *Causal Factors Analysis: An Approach to Organizational Learning* (Hartley et al., 2008).

[10] This is also what we promote in our CFA approach to event investigation.

Index

Index

A

accident vulnerability, *see* practical drift
accidents
    agents and victims, 13
    cause, 147
    industrial, 21, 110
    models of, 146
    see also individual accidents; system accidents
accommodational corrective actions, 115–116
active errors
    described, 102
    prevention of, 102–103
    vs. latent errors, 92
administrative defenses, 93, 103
anticipation of the unexpected, 47, 48–51
artifacts, organizational culture and, 123, 124, 167–168
assumptions, organizational culture and, 123–124, 125, 167–168

B

Barrier Analysis
    evaluation matrix, 138, 139–140
    flawed defenses and, 143–144, 146, 147
barriers to system accidents
    Barrier Analysis matrix, 138, 139–140
    employee knowledge and verification of, 137–138
    escalation of problems and, 16
    failure of, 90–93, 105, 125, 143–144
    flawed defenses and, 143–144, 146, 147
    management of, 103–106, 138
    redundancy and, 21
beliefs and values, organizational culture and, 123, 124, 167–168
benchmarking of best practices, 149–150

Break-the-Chain Framework
overview, 29, 42–43, 96–97
consequence identification, 97–98
defense management, 103–106
event investigations (Causal Factors Analysis), 143–147
fire safety example, 111–113
hazard identification and minimization, 98–101
hazard vulnerability reduction, 106–107
human performance error precursors and, 101–103
illustrations of, 83, 97, 135, 145
industrial safety example, 110–111
lessons to be learned (LTBL), 118–119
pitfalls leading to system accidents, 82–96
safety system evaluation, 113
steps to break the chain, 96–109
tiered approach to learning, 135–150
TWIN Analysis matrix and, 102, 104, 138–139
verification of, 135–136
work-as-imagined vs. work-as-done, 108–109

C

catastrophes
and becoming an HRO, 8–10
complacency and system accidents, 84–85
system failures and, 7
Causal Analysis Handbook (TXU), 101
Causal Factors Analysis (event investigation tool)
overview, 143–144
employee behavior and, 123
flowchart, 148
HRO attribute evaluation and, 44, 144–147
organizational weakness determination, 144
output for HRO attribute evaluation, 145
process steps and flowchart, 147–148
Causal Factors Analysis (Hartley et al.), 145, 147, 188
ceremonial or political corrective actions, 116
characteristic physical items, organizational culture and, 165–166
chronic unease

external event case studies and, 149–150
hazard identification and, 83, 85–86, 99
mindfulness and, 46, 49
safety culture and, 125, 128–129
collective assumptions, *see* organizational culture
Columbia shuttle accident, 9–10, 142
commitment to resilience, 46, 50, 51
common-mode failure, 18, 20
communication
culture of reliability and, 121
norms and, 163
organizational weakness and, 154
safety culture and, 39
supervisor-employee feedback importance, 28, 43, 67, 132, 136–140
systems management and, 24, 28, 139, 189
complacency
accident rarity and, 39, 84, 149–150
hazard identification and, 99
human nature and, 90, 95–96, 104
mindfulness and, 49, 98
redundant barriers and, 21
safety culture and, 117–126
system accidents and, 83, 84–85, 149–150
complex interactivity
hazard identification and minimization, 100–101
redundancy and, 20
unplanned events and, 17–18
component interdependence, 17–19
Conduct of Operations philosophy, 68
consequences
D-words, 13
identification and prioritization, 97–98
reduction and mitigation, 106
Corcoran, William R.
Barrier Analysis matrix, 139
on importance of safety culture, 157
on lessons to be learned, 119
on lowering expectations, 115
on management transparency, 30

on organizational culture characterization, 161

on positive control, 40, 102–103

on system accidents and disasters, 13

corrective actions

accommodational, 115–116

ceremonial or political, 116

effectiveness verification, 114, 119–120

fundamental, 117

human error and, 117–118

monitoring results, 63–64

safety culture and, 157

symptomatic, 116–117

culture of reliability (HRO Practice 3)

overview, 29–30, 39, 122

characterization of, 160–166

evaluation of HRO practice effectiveness, 152–153, 153, 166–168

fostering of, 29–30, 39–40, 43–44, 50, 126–130, 179–180

hazard vulnerability reduction and, 106–107

health of, 167–168, 184–186

knowledge theory and, 190

lines of inquiry into HRO practices, 168–170

organizational learning and adaptation, 30–32, 51, 147–150

performance evaluation metrics, 170–171

system management and, 172–175

see also safety system

D

D-words (system accident consequences), 13

data evaluation

event comparison, 152

HRO practice effectiveness evaluation, 152–153, 153

level of significance, 150–151

singular event extrapolation, 151–152

decision making

consistent conservatism of, 126–127

decentralization of, 107, 126–127

feedback interpretation and integration and, 150–152, 153

hands-on work proficiency and, 127–128

defense management
Break-the-Chain Framework and, 103–106
Causal Factors Analysis and, 145
defenses-in-depth redundancy, 21, 83, 90–93, 103, 105, 149
deference to expertise, 46, 50
Dekker, Sidney
on accident models, 146
on cause, 147
on deviations from the norm, 135
on safety, 138
on safety culture, 152
on stress consequences, 140
on understanding errors, 141
on work-as-imagined vs. work-as-done, 141
Deming, W. E.
on knowledge of knowledge, 30–31
on knowledge of psychology, 126
on knowledge of systems, 27–28, 38, 40, 46, 135
on knowledge of variation, 29, 150, 153
on overall management, 139
on prediction and management, 131
Theory of Profound Knowledge, 24–27, 159, 189–191

E

ECAQ (extraneous conditions adverse to quality), 114, 147
education and training of employees, 65–66, 126–128
employees
complacency and, 125–126
culture of reliability and, 29–30, 43–44
hands-on work proficiency, 127–128
hazard vulnerability reduction, 106–107
training and education, 65–66, 126–128
unsafe acts and, 94–96
engineered defenses, 91–93, 103, 105
errors
active vs. latent, 92
performance modes and error rates, 87–89
precursors, 89–90, 91

reduction of individual, 97, 101–103

system accidents and, 83, 89–90

espoused beliefs and values, organizational culture and, 123, 124, 167–168

events

Causal Factors Analysis of, 150–154

escalation of, 18–19, 86

external, 147–150

investigation of, 143–144

unplanned, 9, 11, 18–19, 100

see also system accidents; system events

expertise, deference to, 46, 50

extraneous conditions adverse to quality (ECAQ), 114, 147

F

fallibility, *see* human error

Federal Aviation Agency (FAA), 82

feedback generation

overview, 132–133

Break-the-Chain Framework verification (Tier 0), 135–136

supervisor-employee communication (Tier 1), 136–140

routine monitoring (Tier 2), 140–143

event investigations (Tier 3), 143–147

external event case studies (Tier 4), 147–150

feedback loops and, 133–134, 150–152, 153

organizational weakness identification, 154–155

refinement of HRO practices and, 153–157

reporting and feedback mechanisms, 31–32, 39–40, 63, 108–109

feedback loops, organizational learning and, 133–134, 150–152, 153

flawed defenses, 143–144, 145, 146, 147

formality of operations philosophy, 68

fostering culture of reliability (HRO Practice 3)

overview, 29–30

lines of inquiry and suggested metrics, 179–180

management roles, 39–40, 43–44, 126–130

mindfulness and, 50

fundamental corrective actions, 117

G

gap analysis
> best practices benchmarking and, 149–150
> Company Alpha example, 70–76
> described, 56, 57
> strategy modification and, 60

Grenoble, Dr. Skip, 151

H

hazardous materials
> catastrophe prevention and, 7, 40–41, 85–86
> system accidents and, 85–86

hazardous operations, *see* high-hazard operations

hazards
> defined, 14
> consequences associated with, 41–42
> identification and minimization of, 83, 85–86, 98–101, 145, 148
> vulnerability reduction, 106–107

high-hazard operations
> hazard vulnerability reduction, 10, 41–43, 106–107
> HRO transformation, 8–10
> management commitment to HRO transformation, 32–33, 74–75
> mindfulness and, 45–46, 98
> operational risk factors overview, 16–22
> pitfalls leading to system accidents, 82–96
> safety system management and, 40–41
> susceptibility to system accidents, 22

high reliability organization (HRO), *see* HRO; HRO practices; HRO transformation

HPI (Human Performance Improvement) process, 97, 101–103

HPI+ process, 97, 101–103, 108, 176, 177

HRO (high reliability organization)
> defined, 7–8
> corrective action programs, 63–64
> "roadmap" to Volume 1 manual, 34–35
> sustaining characteristics of, 46–48
> system accident prevention effectiveness, 141–143

systems approach overview, 23–26
systems approach to HRO transformation planning, 54–58

HRO practices
Break-the-Chain Framework and, 97
Causal Factors Analysis evaluation of, 144–147
fostering culture of reliability, 29–30, 39–40, 43–44, 50, 126–130, 179–180
knowledge theory framework for, 26–27
McKinsey 7S planning approach to, 58
mindful approach to, 44–46
organizational learning, 30–32, 51, 147–150, 182–183
strategy development and, 68, 149–150
sustaining over time, 33, 37–38, 45, 192
system management, 27–28, 48, 172–175
system variability reduction, 29, 49, 153–158, 176–178
see also culture of reliability

HRO transformation
overview, 8–10, 55–57
management commitment to, 32–33, 74–75, 193
McKinsey 7S planning approach, 58–68, 192
McKinsey 7S planning approach example (Company Alpha), 68–80
resource allocation and, 61–62
see also feedback generation; organizational learning

human error
Company Alpha example, 73
corrective actions and, 117–118
fallibility and catastrophes, 7
HRO strategies and, 59
redundancy as management tool, 19–21
system accidents and, 83, 86–89, 148

Human Error (Reason), 86–87

human nature
human performance error precursors and, 90
TWIN Analysis matrix and, 102, 104, 138–139

human performance error precursors
Causal Factors Analysis and, 144, 145, 145–146, 147
human nature and, 90
recognition and reduction of, 101–104, 149
system accidents and, 83, 89–90, 94
see also TWIN Analysis

Index 211

Human Performance Fundamentals (INPO), 101
Human Performance Improvement (HPI) process, error reduction and, 97,
  101–103

I

In Search of Excellence (Peters and Waterman), 55
independent redundancy, 20
individual accidents
  Break-the-Chain Framework and, 103, 110–111
  safety system and, 40, 41
  versus system accidents, 13, 14–16
individual capabilities, 90, 104
individual error, *see* human error
industrial safety, 21, 103, 110
information-rich events, 143, 147
institutions, organizational culture and, 164–165
interactive complexity
  hazard identification and minimization, 100–101
  redundancy and, 20
  unplanned events and, 17–18
interdependence of components, 17–19

K

knowledge-based human errors, 87, 88–89
knowledge theory
  overview, 24–26
  as framework for HRO practices, 26–27
  knowledge of knowledge, 30–32, 191
  knowledge of psychology, 30, 126, 190
  knowledge of systems, 27–28, 38, 40, 46, 135, 189
  knowledge of variation, 29, 150, 153, 190

L

LaPorte and Consolini, 7
latent conditions
  Causal Factors Analysis and, 144
  defense management and, 91–92

latent organizational weakness
   Causal Factors Analysis and, 145, 146
   management control processes and, 94–96
learning, *see* feedback generation
lessons to be learned (LTBL)
   Causal Factors Analysis results and, 147
   observed behavioral changes and, 118–119
   safety culture and, 156
line supervisors, employee communications and, 137–138
linear interactions, unplanned events and, 17–18
lines of inquiry for HRO practice evaluation
   overview, 168–170
   culture of reliability fostering, 179–180
   organizational learning and adaptation, 182–183
   system management, 172–175
   system variability reduction, 176–178
LTBL (lessons to be learned)
   Causal Factors Analysis results and, 147
   observed behavioral changes and, 118–119
   safety culture and, 156

M

management
   commitment to HRO transformation, 32–33, 74–75
   control process deficiencies, 94–96
   culture of reliability and, 29–30
   knowledge theory and, 24–26
   system accidents and, 63, 91–93
management expectations, *see* work-as-imagined vs. work-as-done
managers
   Break-the-Chain Framework implementation, 108–109
   employee communications, 136–140
   fostering culture of reliability and, 39–40, 43–44, 126–130
   problem solving approaches, 156–158
   staff training and recognition, 65–66
   style and leadership, 39, 67–68, 129–130, 185
   system management actions overview, 38
   transparency of leadership, 30, 39

Index   **213**

Managing the Unexpected (Weick and Sutcliffe), 45
McKinsey 7S planning approach
    overview, 54–55
    HRO practices and strategy development, 68
    latent organizational weaknesses and, 152, 154–155
    shared value element, 59
    skills element, 66
    staff element, 65–66
    strategy element, 59–62
    structure element, 64–65
    style element, 67–68
    system element, 62–64
McKinsey 7S planning approach example (Company Alpha)
    company overview, 68–70
    gap analysis, 70–76
    initiative identification, 77–78
    measure tracking, 78
    shared value establishment, 70
    strategies, measures, and targets summary, 79–80
    strategy development and modification for gap closure, 76–77
    strategy measures and annual target development, 77
metrics for performance evaluation
    overview, 170–171
    culture of reliability fostering and, 179–180
    organizational learning and adaptation, 182–183
    system management and, 172–175
    system variability reduction and, 176–178
mindful approach to HRO practices (Weick and Sutcliffe)
    overview, 23, 45–47
    culture of reliability and, 50
    organizational learning and, 51
    sustaining characteristics of, 46–48
    system management and, 48
    system variability reduction and, 49
    work-as-imagined vs. work-as-done, 94–96
modes of error, 87–89

N

Normal Accident Theory (Perrow), 23, 46, 62
normal accidents, *see* system accidents
normalized deviance, 84–85
norms, organizational culture and, 162–164

O

obtaining information, *see* feedback generation
on-the-ground operations, *see* work-as-imagined vs. work-as-done
open systems perspective on organizational function, 10–11
operational success, 8–9, 22, 30–32
organizational accidents, *see* system accidents
organizational attributes, organizational culture and, 123, 124
organizational culture
    overview, 122–125
    changes to, 184–186
    characteristic physical items, 165–166
    characterization of, 160–166
    collective assumptions, 123–124, 125
    Company Alpha example, 75
    importance of, 126
    insights to, 147
    institutions, 164–165
    management style and leadership, 67–68, 129–130, 185
    model of, 123–124
    norms, 162–164
    shared mental content, 161–162
    system accidents and, 94–96
    underlying assumptions, 123–124, 125, 167–168
    unwritten rules and, 156
    see also safety culture
organizational function systems perspective, 10–11
organizational harm, 7
organizational learning (HRO Practice 4)
    Company Alpha example, 74
    external event case studies, 147–150
    feedback integration and interpretation, 150–152, 153

interactive complexity and tight coupling, 100

knowledge theory and, 191

lessons to be learned and, 118–119

lines of inquiry and suggested metrics, 182–183

mindfulness and, 51

PDCA cycle, 31–32

process start-up verification and, 135–136

safety system management and, 44

systematic process adjustment and, 113

see also Break-the-Chain Framework; culture of reliability; feedback generation

organizational transformation, *see* HRO transformation

organizational weaknesses

common, 154–155

determination of, 143–144

latent, 151–152

P

PDCA (planning, doing, checking, and acting) cycle, 31–32

performance data, routine monitoring of, 140–143

performance modes of human error, 87–89

Perrow, Charles

on inevitability of system accidents, 17, 32

on interactive complexity and tight coupling, 17–18, 100

Normal Accident Theory, 23, 46, 62

on redundancy, 20–21

Phoenix Handbook (Corcoran), 119

pitfalls leading to system accidents

Break-the-Chain Framework and, 82–83

complacency and, 84–85

defense management and, 91–93

hazard recognition and, 85–86

human error threats and, 86–89

human performance error precursors and, 89–90

work-as-imagined vs. work-as-done, 94–96

planning, doing, checking, and acting (PDCA) cycle, 31–32

positive control, 40, 102–103

practical drift

defined, 9
organizational susceptibility to, 9, 22
prevention of, 39
redundancy and, 21
system accidents and, 83, 85–86, 94–95
preoccupation with failure, 46, 49
problem solving, systems thinking approach to, 156–158
professed culture, organizational culture and, 123, 124

R

Reason, Dr. James
on accident causes, 94–95
on defenses-in-depth, 92
on human error, 86–87, 89, 102
on organizational weakness determination, 144
on outcome data and system safety, 141
redundancy
overview, 19
defenses-in-depth, 21, 83, 91–93, 103, 105
independent redundancy, 20
negative aspects of, 20–21
practical drift and, 21
system opacity and, 21
reliability, 8, 59
reluctance to simplify, 46, 48
resilience, commitment to, 46, 50, 51
Rickover, Admiral Hyman G., 39, 40, 41, 44
Roberts, Karlene, 8
routine monitoring, 132, 140–143
rule-based human errors, 87, 88

S

safety
defined, 8
HRO status and, 59
industrial, 21, 103, 110
safety basis and safe operations, 14

safety culture
     complacency and, 125–126
     defined, 39
     of FAA, 82
     importance of, 153, 156
safety records
     commercial airlines and HRO status, 8
     nuclear power plants and HRO status, 8–9
     outcome data and system safety, 141–142
     practical drift and, 9
safety system
     corrective action implementation, 114–119
     corrective measure verification, 119–120
     decentralized decision making and, 126–127
     ensuring provision of safety and, 39, 40–41
     evaluation of, 113, 128–130
     hands-on work proficiency and, 127–128
     infrastructure maintenance and, 127
     organizational learning and, 44
     systematic process adjustment, 113
     variability reduction, 41–43
Sagan, Scott D., 11, 23
Schein, Dr. Edgar, 122–124, 129, 151, 184–185
sensitivity to operations, 46, 51
7S planning approach, *see* McKinsey 7S planning approach
shared mental content, organizational culture and, 167–168
shared value (7S planning element), 55–56, 59, 70
skill-based human errors, 87, 88
skills (7S planning element), 66, 74
staff (7S planning element), 65–66, 75–76
strategy (7S planning element), 59–62, 76–80
The Strategy-Focused Organization (Kaplan and Norton), 60–61
structure (7S planning element), 64–65, 70–71
style (7S planning element), 67–68, 74–75
symptomatic corrective actions, 116–117
system (7S planning element), 62–64, 71–74
system accidents
     defined, 11–12, 14
     barriers to, 16, 21

commonalities of, 150
complex interactions and, 18
consequences (D-words), 13
examples of, 14, 32
prevention of, 41–43, 59, 103
redundant barriers and, 21
versus individual accidents, 13, 14–16
system accidents, pitfalls leading to
Break-the-Chain Framework, 82–83
complacency, 84–85
defense management, 91–93
hazard recognition, 85–86
human error threats, 86–89
human performance error precursors, 89–90
work-as-imagined vs. work-as-done, 94–96
system coupling, event escalation and, 18–19
system events, 12–13
system failures, 7
system management (HRO Practice 1)
overview, 37–40
culture of reliability and, 43–44
knowledge theory and, 27–28, 189
leadership and, 44
lines of inquiry and suggested metrics, 172–175
mindfulness and, 44–48
safety system and, 40–43
system variability reduction (HRO Practice 2)
knowledge theory and, 29, 190
lines of inquiry and suggested metrics, 176–178
mindfulness and, 49
systems approach to, 153, 156–158
see also Break-the-Chain Framework
systems
characteristics of, 12
defined, 10
integrity of, 16
redundancy and, 21
systems perspective on organizational function, 10–11
systems thinking approach to problem solving, 156–158

T

tasks
>manager expectations and, 137
>performance modes and error rates, 87–89
>task demand error precursors, 89–90, 102
>TWIN Analysis matrix, 104

Theory of Profound Knowledge (Deming), 24–27, 159, 189–191

threat, 14

tightly coupled systems
>event escalation and, 18–19
>hazard identification and minimization, 100–101
>system accidents and, 85–86

training and education
>employee decision making and, 126–128
>hands-on work proficiency, 127–128

transformation, *see* HRO transformation

TWIN Analysis
>described, 102
>Causal Factors Analysis and, 144, 145, 145–146
>human performance error precursor identification, 102, 104, 138–139

U

underlying assumptions
>Company Omega example, 125
>organizational culture and, 123–124, 167–168

unhealthy safety culture, 167–168, 184–186

unplanned events, 9, 11, 17–19, 100

unsafe acts
>Causal Factors Analysis and, 144
>organizational culture and, 95–96

V

variability reduction
>knowledge theory and, 29
>mindfulness and, 49
>safety system management and, 41–43
>systems approach to HRO refinement, 153, 156–158

Vaughan, Diane, 84–85
victims, accident, 13

W

Weick, Karl, and Kathleen Sutcliffe, 23, 45–47, 48–51, 192–193
work-as-imagined vs. work-as-done
    Break-the-Chain Framework implementation, 108–109
    Causal Factors Analysis and, 145, 147
    manager-employee communication and, 140
    perceived gaps in, 141
    system accidents and, 83, 94–96, 149
work environment
    human performance error precursors and, 90
    TWIN Analysis matrix and, 102, 104, 138–1395

Z

Zebroski, Edwin L., 150